Echocardiographic Diagnosis of Cardiac Malformations

Echocardiographic Diagnosis of Cardiac Malformations

Roberta G. Williams, M.D.
Associate Professor of Pediatrics, University of California, Los Angeles, UCLA School of Medicine; Chief, Department of Pediatrics, Division of Cardiology, UCLA Medical Center, University of California, Los Angeles, UCLA School of Medicine, Los Angeles, California

Fredrick Z. Bierman, M.D.
Assistant Professor, Columbia University College of Physicians and Surgeons; Director, Pediatric Cardiac Ultrasound, Columbia-Presbyterian Medical Center, New York, New York

Stephen P. Sanders, M.D.
Assistant Professor of Pediatrics, Harvard Medical School; Director, Cardiac Non-Invasive Laboratory, The Children's Hospital, Boston, Massachusetts

LITTLE, BROWN AND COMPANY, BOSTON/TORONTO

Library of Congress Catalog Card No. 86-80369

ISBN 0-316-94132-8

Printed in the United States of America

MV

**This book is dedicated
to our families and
to Dr. Alexander Nadas**

Contents

Preface   *ix*
Acknowledgments   *xi*
Introduction   *1*

PART I
IMAGING THE
NORMAL HEART

1. Precordial Imaging   *4*

2. Subxiphoid Approach   *14*

3. Suprasternal Approach   *27*

4. Interrelationships of Different Views   *29*

PART II
SHUNT LESIONS

5. Atrial Septal Defect   *36*

6. Ventricular Septal Defect   *51*

7. Complete Atrioventricular Canal Defects   *63*

8. Patent Ductus Arteriosus   *71*

9. Total Anomalous Pulmonary Venous Connection   *74*

10. Partial Anomalous Pulmonary Venous Connection   *84*

11. Aorticopulmonary Window   *86*

12. Anomalous Left Coronary Artery   *89*

PART III
OBSTRUCTIVE
LESIONS

13. Ebstein's Anomaly of the Tricuspid Valve   *94*

14. Tricuspid Atresia   *99*

15. Hypoplastic Right Heart: Critical Pulmonic Stenosis and Pulmonary
    Atresia with Intact Ventricular Septum   *103*

16. Double-Chambered Right Ventricle   *108*

17. Valvar Pulmonary Stenosis   *111*

18. Congenital Mitral Obstruction   *113*

19. Cor Triatriatum   *118*

20. Hypoplastic Left Heart Syndrome: Mitral and Aortic Atresia   *121*

21. Fixed Left Ventricular Outflow Obstruction   *127*

22. Hypertrophic Cardiomyopathy   *132*

23. Valvar Aortic Stenosis   *137*

24. Coarctation of the Aorta   *142*

25. Interrupted Aortic Arch   *146*

PART IV
CONOTRUNCAL
ABNORMALITIES

26. General Features of Conotruncal Abnormalities   *152*

27. Tetralogy of Fallot   *155*

28. Absent Pulmonary Valve Syndrome (with Tetralogy of Fallot)   *163*

29. Simple or D-Transposition of the Great Arteries   *165*

30. Corrected or L-Transposition of the Great Arteries   *170*

31. Double Outlet Right Ventricle   *178*

32. Truncus Arteriosus   *184*

PART V
COMPLEX HEART
DISEASE

33. Heterotaxy Syndrome: A Segmental Approach to the Diagnosis of Congenital Heart Defects   *188*

34. Single Ventricle   *199*

35. Straddling Atrioventricular Valves   *204*

36. Juxtaposition of the Atrial Appendages   *208*

37. Cardiac Malpositions   *211*

PART VI
EVALUATION OF
POSTOPERATIVE
PATIENTS

38. Evaluation of Postoperative Patients   *214*

Index   *229*

Preface

There must be a thousand better things to do than to write another book on echocardiography, and yet, after an interminable number of lost weekends, *Echocardiographic Diagnosis of Cardiac Malformations* has taken on its final form. The impetus for this task has been the need to set forth a concept for approaching the diagnosis of congenital cardiac lesions. There are many excellent books providing basic information on the principles of ultrasound and cardiac imaging. They provide a good background for the subject of this book, which emphasizes the diagnostic challenges imposed by the wide anatomic spectrum of cardiac malformations.

The first part describes the many transducer positions and planes used to image the heart and great vessels, with emphasis on similitude of the different approaches. Special attention is given to a discussion of multiple-plane imaging from the subxiphoid (subcostal) position because this technique of imaging has not been previously published in a comprehensive form. Since the subxiphoid approach has proved most valuable in the evaluation of infants, it is emphasized in those chapters describing lesions that frequently present in infancy. Subsequent chapters deal with the anatomy, suggested examination techniques, diagnostic features, and pitfalls within the general categories of shunt lesions, obstructive lesions, conotruncal anomalies, complex lesions, and postoperative studies.

Because we wish this book to be of use to echocardiographers who are not primarily pediatric cardiologists and to pediatric cardiologists who are not echocardiographers, we have dwelt on the finer anatomic points and the technique required to define them within each diagnostic category. Our task was made more difficult by the ever changing terminology. Whenever possible, we have used multiple terminologies with the hope that one phrase, at least, will be familiar to the reader; this has not been carried to the extreme, but only to the degree sufficient to clarify the anatomic principle.

Echocardiographic Diagnosis of Cardiac Malformations focuses on the anatomic diagnosis of cardiac malformations and thus does not address the many contributions of Doppler echocardiography to the physiologic evaluation of these lesions, unless Doppler echocardiography specifically adds to the qualitative diagnosis. It is hoped that the reader will find this book a handy reference as well as a model for a comprehensive approach to the examination of young patients with suspected heart disease.

R. G. W.
F. Z. B.
S. P. S.

Acknowledgments

The authors are indebted to many people who provided the environment in which this book was created. Dr. Alexander Nadas gave each of us our start and provided a competitive, questioning environment that stimulated clinical excellence and attracted the large and diverse patient population that provides the basis for this book. Dr. Richard Van Praagh and Dr. Stella Van Praagh imbued us with an understanding of anatomic concepts and an abiding appreciation for the vast scope of complex cardiac morphology. Dr. Aldo Castaneda pushed back the frontiers of age and complexity in the repair of congenital lesions, forcing us to provide a comprehensive diagnosis and stimulating us to methodically examine our mistakes and to learn from them. We have continued to learn the surgical relevance of echocardiographic findings from our productive associations with Dr. Hillel Laks and Dr. William Norwood. Dr. Kenneth Fellows provided thoughtful and high-quality angiographic interpretations for comparison with our studies and joined us in exploring the best complementary uses of the two techniques.

The authors are pleased and grateful for the professionalism and precision of anatomic detail of Gwynne Gloege in the production of the artwork for this book.

Several generations of secretaries gave generously their effort and peace of mind to produce the multiple revisions and last-minute chapter additions: Barbara Cesaro, Carrol Cohen, and Kathleen O'Brien.

The authors are particularly indebted to the staff of Little, Brown and Company, who showed great patience and understanding to authors struggling with time and space.

Special thanks go to our families for their forbearance.

Introduction

The echocardiographic diagnosis of congenital heart disease is challenging because of the limitless variations of cardiac anatomy and the need to define all extracardiac structures such as great arteries and veins as well as all intracardiac structures. These structures must be displayed in multiple planes in order to define a complex shape (e.g., interventricular septum) in three dimensions and to describe both absolute and relative positional information. These special problems stimulated the development of the method for multiple-plane imaging of the heart and great vessels described herein.

The subxiphoid (also known as subcostal) approach has proved most flexible for imaging the heart and great vessels in the infant and young child. Initially, this approach was selected because it places the heart of the infant at an optimal distance from the transducer and thus avoids the problem of beam convergence in the near field of a sector format. By angling, rotating, and moving the transducer in the subxiphoid and right and left subcostal positions, the heart and great vessels can be viewed in an infinite variety of planes. The development of longer-focused transducers has facilitated the subxiphoid approach in larger patients and has provided good lateral resolution of structures within the posterior and superior mediastinum in patients of all sizes.

This book is primarily concerned with the complete anatomic diagnosis of the infant or child with congenital heart disease. Although all pertinent views will be discussed, there will be an emphasis on the subxiphoid approach because it has been most useful in examining younger patients. Since multiple-plane imaging from the subxiphoid position has not been previously described in its entirety, it will be thoroughly discussed here, along with the relative merits of other views.

Imaging the Normal Heart

CHAPTER 1

Precordial Imaging

*Parasternal Long-
Axis View*

The *parasternal long-axis view* is aligned in a plane from the ascending aorta to the left ventricular (LV) apex (Fig. 1-1). In infants, the apex of the heart extends more directly leftward than in older patients so that the transducer is aligned more horizontally with respect to the torso. The parasternal long-axis view demonstrates the anteroposterior (A-P) and superior right–inferior left relations of the long axis of the LV outflow tract from apex to aortic root. The length of the outflow tract is displayed, with the outflow ventricular septum forming its anterior border and the length of anterior mitral leaflet forming its posterior border. The subaortic, central, and apical segments of the interventricular septum (IVS) are seen from this view. The membranous and inflow portions of the septum are not seen in this plane unless there is extreme rotation of the heart due to right ventricular (RV) dilation.

*Parasternal Short-
Axis Views*

The *parasternal short-axis views* are at right angles to the parasternal long-axis view and display the A-P and inferior right–superior left coordinates of the LV. Serial short-axis views are obtained by sweeping the transducer from base to apex, displaying sequentially (1) the lengths of the RV outflow tract, main pulmonary artery (MPA), and proximal branches as they wrap around the aortic root (Fig. 1-2), (2) cross section of the aortic valve with left atrium (LA) behind (Fig. 1-3), (3) mitral valve orifice and LV outflow tract (Fig. 1-4), and (4) papillary muscles of the LV (Fig. 1-5). These sections display all segments of the IVS as well as the lateral and posterior free walls. However, these views often are not optimal for demonstrating the atrioventricular (A-V) canal (inlet) portion of the IVS because of shadowing from sternum or ribs. This shadowing can be partly avoided by extreme left-lateral decubitus positioning of the patient.

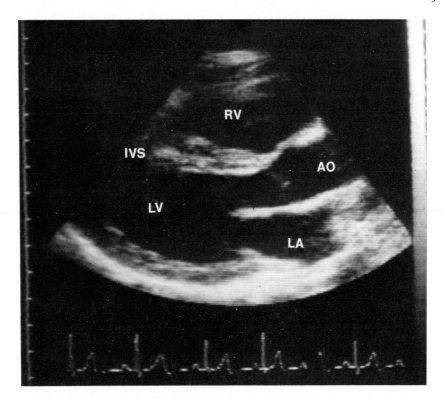

Fig. 1-1. Parasternal long-axis view. The anteroposterior coordinates of the left ventricle (*LV*) are displayed from aortic root (*AO*) to apex. In the normal heart, this view demonstrates continuity between the anterior border of the AO and the subaortic portion of the interventricular septum (*IVS*) and also displays the midmuscular IVS. The apical portion of the IVS is cut off in this frame. *LA* = left atrium; *RV* = right ventricle.

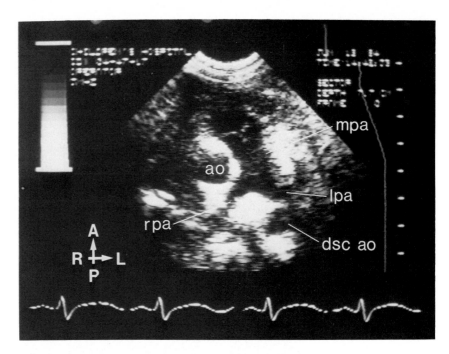

Fig. 1-2. High transverse parasternal view shows the right ventricular outflow tract and main pulmonary artery (*mpa*) and branches. Note how the right pulmonary artery (*rpa*) courses behind the aortic root (*ao*) and the left pulmonary artery (*lpa*) courses posteriorly. Therefore, only the proximal portion of the lpa is seen. *dsc ao* = descending thoracic aorta.

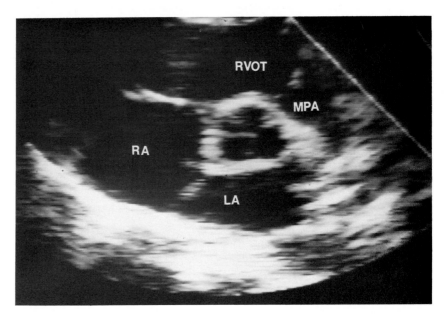

Fig. 1-3. In the transverse parasternal view of the aortic valve, three cusps of the aortic valve are seen within the central circular structure representing the aortic root. The right ventricular outflow tract (*RVOT*) crosses anteriorly. A portion of the main pulmonary artery (*MPA*) is also seen. The right atrium (*RA*) lies to the right of the aorta. The linear structure between RA and RVOT is the tricuspid valve. The left atrium (*LA*) lies directly posterior to the aorta. The linear echoes between the RA and LA represent a portion of the interatrial septum.

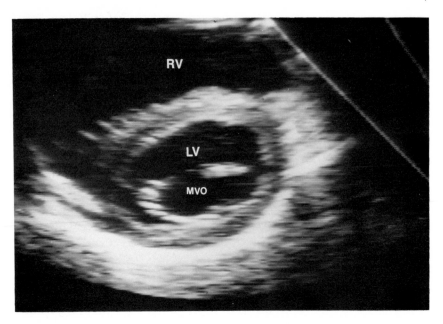

Fig. 1-4. Transverse parasternal view of the midportion of the left ventricle (*LV*) shows the elliptic orifice of the mitral valve (*MVO*). The outflow portion of the LV is anterior to the MVO. The midmuscular portion of the intraventricular septum is viewed here. *RV* = right ventricle.

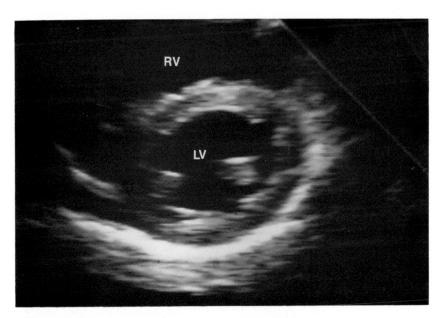

Fig. 1-5. Transverse parasternal view of the left ventricle (*LV*) at the level of the papillary muscles. The area of the interventricular septum viewed here is the lower portion of the midmuscular septum. The apical portion of the septum is displayed by sweeping from this plane toward the apex. *RV* = right ventricle.

Right Parasternal
Views

In some patients, excellent parasternal long- and short-axis views of the LV can be obtained by rolling the patient into a steep right-lateral decubitus position, placing the transducer along the right sternal border, and aiming medially, in equivalent positions, to the left parasternal long- and short-axis views. Imaging success varies from patient to patient because of differences in chest configuration and mobility of the mediastinum.

Aligning the transducer in the parasternal long axis of the LV provides an excellent view of the ascending aorta (Fig. 1-6). Maintaining this angulation while sliding the transducer up toward the right subclavicular area traces the ascending aorta to the transverse arch. In some patients, this technique provides a comprehensive image of the ascending aorta and transverse arch (Fig. 1-7). The right pulmonary artery (RPA) is seen in cross section, nestled in the crook of the aortic arch. The length of the right superior vena cava (SVC) and the interatrial septum can be displayed by inclining the transducer slightly to the right of the ascending aorta. Sliding or angling the transducer inferiorly demonstrates the junction of the IVC with the right atrium (RA).

Fig. 1-6. Echo displays long axis of aorta (*Ao*) and the left ventricle (*LV*) from a right parasternal long-axis view. This view, obtained by rolling the patient into a steep right-lateral decubitus position, is very similar to the left parasternal long-axis view except that more of the ascending Ao is displayed. As a result, the right parasternal long-axis view is excellent for demonstrating supravalvar aortic stenosis. A more rightward aspect of the interventricular septum is also seen, allowing a view of a perimembranous ventricular septum, which is usually obscured by the sternum in the left parasternal plane. *RV* = right ventricle.

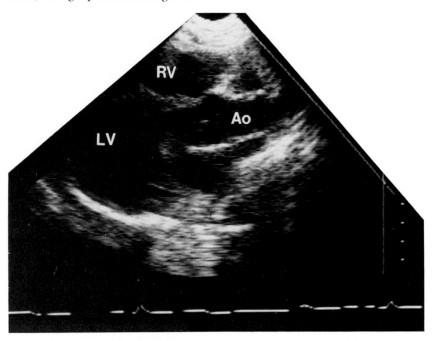

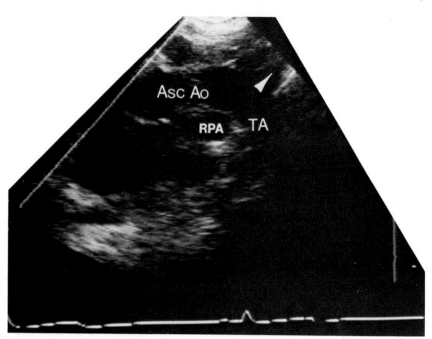

Fig. 1-7. High right parasternal view of typical left aortic arch displays ascending aorta (*Asc Ao*), brachiocephalic vessels (*arrow*) and transverse arch (*TA*). The right pulmonary artery (*RPA*) is seen in cross section. This view is obtained by sliding the transducer superiorly from the right parasternal long-axis position. The plane of the echo beam is almost identical to the plane of the suprasternal notch long-axis view and the intermediate subxiphoid view displayed in Figure 3-1.

Short-axis right sternal–border views are obtained by rotating the transducer 90° to the precordial long axis position. In patients with a good acoustic window, this angle affords an excellent view of the interatrial septum, tricuspid valve, inflow ventricular septum, mitral valve, and even lateral and posterior free walls of the LV (Fig. 1-8). The foramen ovale is nearly perpendicular to the transducer beam, and, as a result, the flap valve of the foramen ovale is clearly displayed. By angling the transducer leftward and inferiorly (similar to short-axis sweeps from the left sternal border), it is possible to obtain cross sections of the LV as seen through the RV. From this vantage point, the inflow ventricular septum is perpendicular to the transducer beam.

Fig. 1-8. Transverse right sternal border view of atria is nearly identical to transverse left sternal border views. The echo beam is nearly perpendicular to the fossa ovalis, resulting in little artifactual dropout. From this position, the transducer may be rotated leftward to obtain cross-sectional views of the ventricles. *Ao* = aorta; *LA* = left atrium; *PA* = pulmonary artery; *RA* = right atrium.

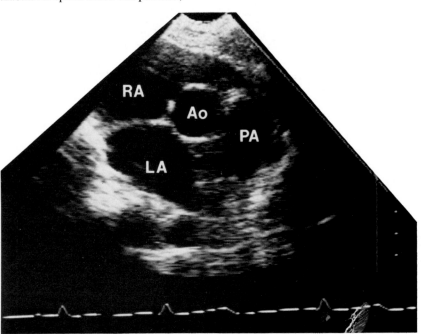

APICAL APPROACH
Apical 4-Chamber View

The *apical 4-chamber view* displays the superoinferior and right-left coordinates of the inflow portions of the two ventricles and the interventricular septum (IVS), the interatrial septum and both atria (Fig. 1-9). This view is useful for displaying the attachments of the atrioventricular (A-V) valve to the crux of the heart, as well as the inflow, central, and apical portions of the IVS. Posterior angulation from the same view displays the coronary sinus (Fig. 1-10). Although limited superior angulation toward the outflow septum may be performed, the outflow septum is not easily viewed from this plane.

Fig. 1-9. This apical 4-chamber view displays the right (*ra*) and left (*la*) atria and inflow portions of the right (*rv*) and left (*lv*) ventricles, with intervening interatrial and interventricular septa and atrioventricular valves.

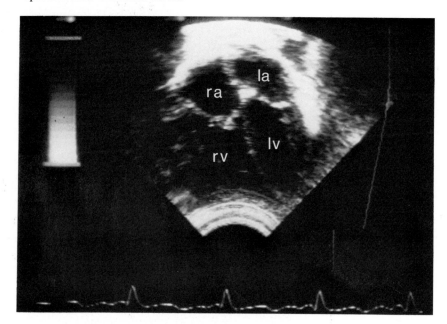

Fig. 1-10. This posteriorly angled apical 4-chamber view displays the coronary sinus (*cs*). *lv* = left ventricle; *ra* = right atrium; *rv* = right ventricle.

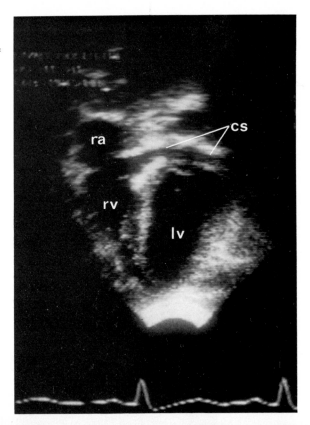

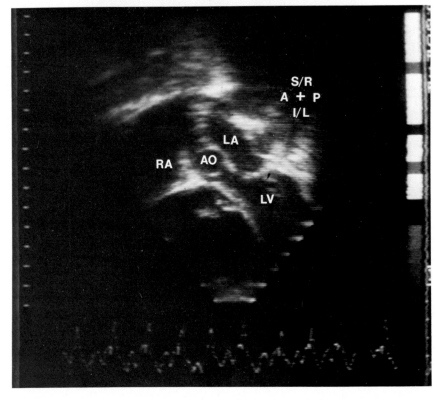

Fig. 1-11. The apical 2-chamber view is nearly identical to the parasternal long-axis view, displaying the long axis of the left ventricular (*LV*) outflow tract from the perspective of the apex. *Ao* = aorta; *LA* = left atrium; *RA* = right atrium.

Dropout of echoes from the interatrial septum and IVS may be artifactual because the surfaces of these structures are nearly parallel to the ultrasound beam.

Apical 2-Chamber View

The *apical 2-chamber view* is nearly in the same plane as the parasternal long-axis view: The same cardiac segments are displayed (Fig. 1-11), but the echo beam is now parallel to the left ventricular (LV) long axis.

The following bibliography pertains to Chapters 1 through 4.

BIBLIOGRAPHY

Popp, R. L., Fowles, R., Coltard, J., et al. Cardiac anatomy viewed systematically with two-dimensional echocardiography. *Chest* 75:579, 1979.

Sahn, D. J., Allen, H. D., McDonald, G., et al. Real time cross-sectional echocardiographic-angiographic correlations. *Circulation* 56:762, 1977.

Schapira, J. N., Martin, R. P., Fowles, R. E., et al. Single and two dimensional echocardiographic features of the interatrial septum in normal subjects and patients with atrial septal defect. *Am. J. Cardiol.* 43:816, 1979.

Schiller, N. B., and Snider, A. R. Echocardiography in congenital heart disease: Key references. *Circulation* 63:461, 1981.

Silverman, N. S., et al. Anatomical basis of cross sectional echocardiography. *Br. Heart J.* 50:421, 1983.

Silverman, N. S., and Schiller, N. B. Apex echocardiography: A two-dimensional technique for evaluating congenital heart disease. *Circulation* 57:503, 1978.

Singer, A. R., Enderlein, M. A., Teitel, D. F., et al. Two-dimensional echocardiographic determination of aortic and pulmonary artery sizes from infancy to adulthood in normal subjects. *Am. J. Cardiol.* 53:218, 1984.

Snider, A. R., and Silverman, N. H. Suprasternal notch echocardiography: A two-dimensional technique for evaluating congenital heart disease. *Circulation* 63:165, 1981.

Tajik, A. J., Seward, J. B., Hagler, D. J., et al. Two-dimensional real-time ultrasonic imaging of the heart and great vessels: Technique, image orientation, structure identification and validation. *Mayo Clin. Proc.* 53:271, 1978.

Subxiphoid Approach

THE NORMAL
SUBXIPHOID
EXAMINATION

In the normal subxiphoid examination, best visualization is achieved with the transducer placed directly beneath the xiphoid process. The transducer is moved to right or left subcostal positions to accommodate variations in cardiac position or produce specific angulation effects.

Although a multitude of transducer positions are possible, subxiphoid imaging of the normal heart may be simplified to two sweeps in orthogonal planes (Fig. 2-1A to C). In the first sweep, the scan plane is oriented parallel to the long axis of the left ventricle (LV) and inclined from inferior vena cava (IVC) to right ventricle (RV). These are called *long-axis views* (Fig.

Fig. 2-1. Three frequently used sub-xiphoid transducer positions. The plane of the echo beam is aligned in the left ventricular long axis (A), the left ventricular short axis (B), and an intermediate position (C), useful for viewing a left aortic arch.

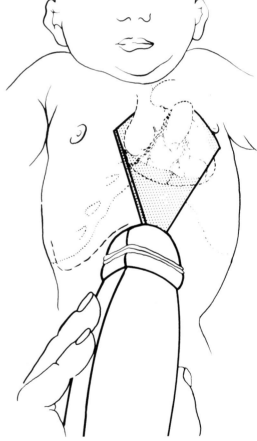

A

2-2). The sweep begins perpendicular to the trunk, displaying the IVC in cross section (Fig. 2-3A,B). The coordinates displayed are anteroposterior (A-P) and right-left. The transducer is then angled superiorly, successively displaying the lower atria, ventricular inflow, ventricular outflow, and finally a coronal view of the anterior ventricle (Figs. 2-4A to C, 2-5A, B, 2-6A to C, 2-7A to C). In the latter extreme superior position, the coordinates displayed are superoinferior and right-left. Thus, the long-axis sweep begins with a horizontal plane, relative to the torso, and ends in an almost coronal plane.

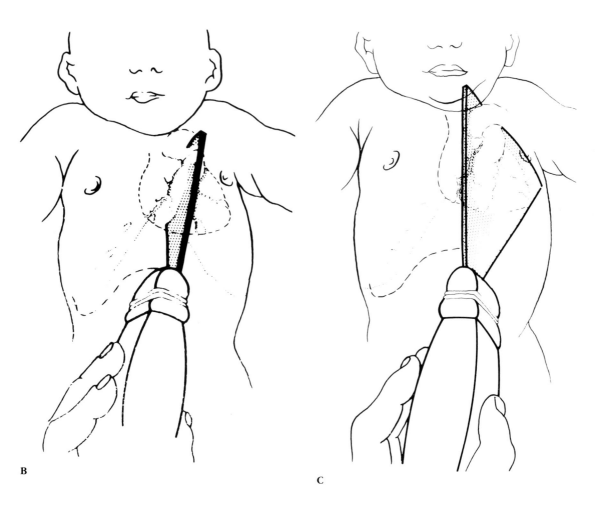

B

C

CHAPTER 2. Subxiphoid Approach

Fig. 2-2. Diagram of the heart, displayed from the right side, demonstrates the subxiphoid long-axis planes. The sweep begins by pointing the transducer toward the liver, with the sector plane perpendicular to the trunk in order to observe the inferior vena cava in cross section. The transducer is then angled superiorly across the floor of the right atrium just above to the entrance of the inferior vena cava. The transducer sweep is continued superiorly to encounter successively more superior and anterior structures within the heart and mediastinum. Although a myriad of views may be obtained, they have been condensed into four planes: (*1*) the floor of the right atrium, (*2*) mid–left atrium and left ventricular inflow, (*3*) long axis of the left ventricle and ascending aorta, and (*4*) a coronal section of the right ventricle.

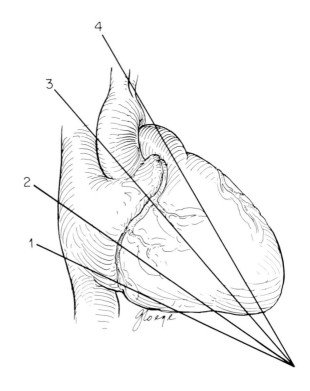

Fig. 2-3. (A) Diagram showing the cross-sectional view of the inferior vena cava (*IVC*) and aorta (*Ao*), which is the initial transducer position in the long-axis sweep. The plane is perpendicular to the torso. Shaded area represents area seen on usual view with IVC to the right and Ao to the left of the spine (*Sp*). (B) Typical echo from area displayed in the diagram revealing the left renal vein (*LRV*) crossing in front of the Ao to join the IVC. Superior mesenteric artery (*SMA*) is also seen.

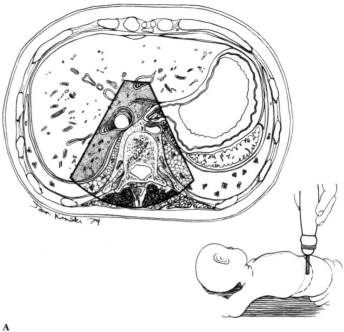

A

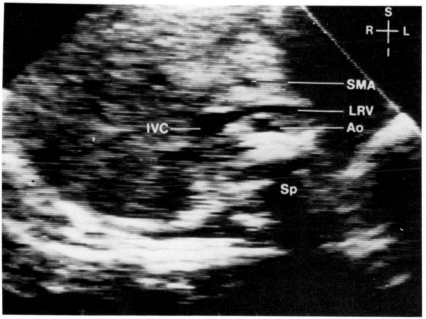

B

CHAPTER 2. Subxiphoid Approach

18

Fig. 2-4. Diagram (A) and echo (B) of subxiphoid (L1) view display the floor of the right (*ra*) and left atria (*LA, la*), the mouth of the coronary sinus (*CS, cs*), the eustachian or right venous valve, the inferior limbic band of the interatrial septum, and the entrance of the lower pulmonary veins (*lpv* and *rpv*) to the la. The last view (C) demonstrates a dilated cs.

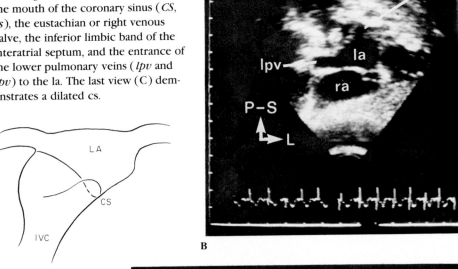

A

B

C

Fig. 2-5. Cut section of dog heart (A) and echo (B) of subxiphoid long-axis plane (corresponding to position 2 in Fig. 2-2), display the midportion of the interatrial septum at the region of the fossa ovalis, the mitral valve, and the long axis of the left ventricle (*lv*) and left ventricular inflow septum (*LVI*). The transducer beam is at a relatively acute angle to the septum primum (*SP*) (flap valve of the foramen ovale), facilitating the display of this thin structure and avoiding artifactual dropout. The right ventricle and tricuspid valve are not usually seen because they are anterior to this plane. *CS* = coronary sinus; *EV* = eustachian valve; *LA, la* = left atrium; *LAA, laa* = left atrial appendage; *lupv* = left upper pulmonary vein; *MA* = mitral annulus; *RA, ra* = right atrium; *RUPV, rupv* = right upper pulmonary vein.

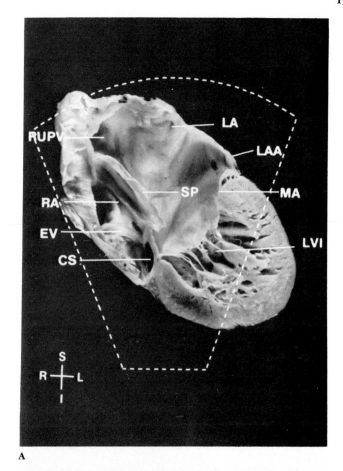

A

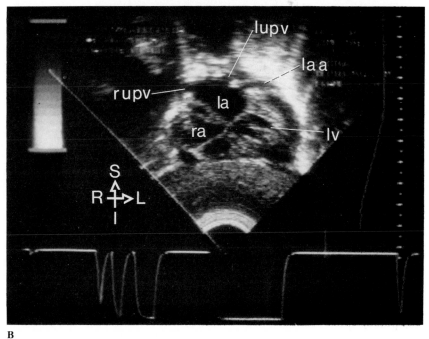

B

CHAPTER 2. Subxiphoid Approach

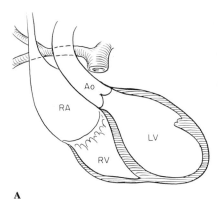

A

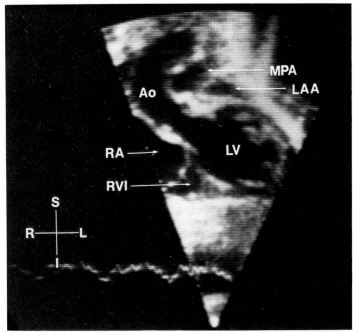

B

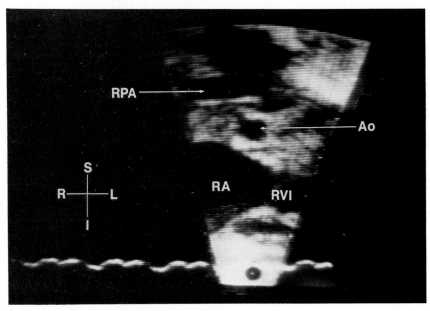

C

Fig. 2-6. Diagram (A) and echo (B) of subxiphoid (L3) view display the long axis of left ventricle (*LV*) and ascending aorta (*Ao*). A partial view of the right ventricular inflow (*RVI*) and tricuspid valve (septal leaflet) is seen. This view is useful for displaying the aortic valve, subaortic area, and the membranous and midmuscular septum. The echo-free space immediately to the left of the main pulmonary artery (*MPA*) repre-sents the left atrial appendage (*LAA*), not a left pulmonary artery. The MPA and right branch pulmonary artery (*RPA*) are demonstrated by pointing the tip of the transducer in a slightly more posterior position than that used in B as seen in frame C. The entire course of the RPA (C) is seen as it runs left to right to cross the superior vena cava. *RA* = right atrium.

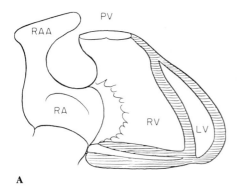

A

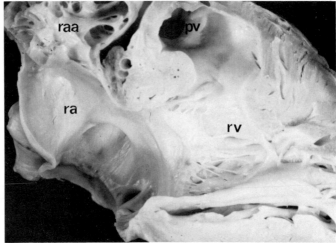

B

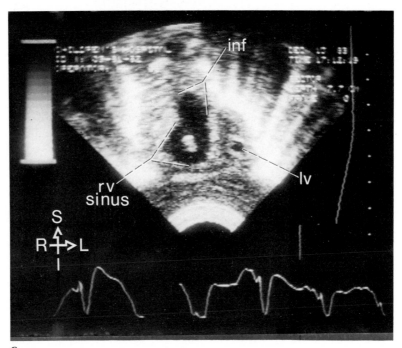

C

Fig. 2-7. Diagram (A), cut section of dog heart (B), and echo (C) demonstrate the subxiphoid long-axis position (L4), a coronal section of the right ventricle (*RV, rv*). This view is obtained by pressing deeply (and gently) into the abdomen and angling the transducer acutely upward. The right-left and superoinferior coordinates of the RV outflow tract as well as the tip of the left ventricle (*LV, lv*) and the anterior muscular septum are displayed. A partial view of the pulmonary cusps at the top of the RV is obtained. *inf* = infundibulum; *PV, pv* = pulmonary vein; *RA, ra* = right atrium; *RAA, raa* = right atrial appendage; *rv sinus* = right ventricular sinus.

CHAPTER 2. Subxiphoid Approach

The second sweep is at right angles to the first; the scan plane is swept perpendicular to the long axis of the LV as the transducer is rotated 90° from the long-axis position and angled from right heart border to apex (Fig. 2-8). The sweep begins in a parasagittal (to the torso) plane, displaying the length of the superior vena cava (SVC) and IVC (Fig. 2-9A, B). The coordinates displayed are A-P and superoinferior. The transducer is angled leftward (and inferiorly if the heart is in a vertical position) to display, successively, midatria, RV inflow, RV outflow, short axis of LV, and LV apex (Figs. 2-10A, B, 2-11A to C, 2-12A, B, 2-13A to C). At the end of the sweep, the transducer points toward the left shoulder.

A left aortic arch is displayed by slight clockwise rotation from a long-axis view that displays the ascending aorta (see Fig. 2-1C). Angulation and rotation from these standard positions (i.e., long- and short-axis views) are required to demonstrate certain anatomic features.

Technical limitations to this approach include abdominal rigidity and gaseous distention, abdominal incisions or defects, and mediastinal chest tubes. During the course of the examination, air tends to be pushed out of the beam path by the transducer so that images may improve with persistence.

Sedation of a young infant is rarely required, as simple distraction or use of a pacifier or bottle is often adequate, but is usually necessary for examination of older infants and toddlers, particularly when Doppler studies are included.

Although the subxiphoid approach is best suited for the infant, development of more sensitive transducers with longer focal ranges has allowed this

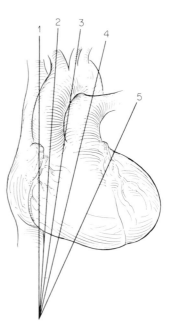

Fig. 2-8. A diagram of the anterior aspect of the heart shows the transverse or short-axis views as the beam plane is oriented perpendicular to the long axis of the left ventricle and swept from right to left. Plane 1 intersects the long axes of the superior and inferior vena cavae as they enter the right atrium. Plane 2 displays the mid–interatrial septum (orthogonal to the midatrial plane of the long-axis sweep, subxiphoid L2). Plane 3 intersects the inflow portion of the right ventricle and the tricuspid valve orifice as well as the left ventricular outflow tract. Plane 4 intersects the long axis of right ventricle and the short axis of the left ventricle at the level of the anterior mitral leaflet. As the transducer sweeps further leftward, a true equatorial cross section of the left ventricle at the level of the papillary muscles is obtained (plane 5).

approach to be used in older children and many adults. The essential requirement is to have the transducer beam focused at the level of interest. In the term newborn, the necessary focal range is approximately from 3 (near atrial and ventricular structures) to 12 cm (aortic arch and superior mediastinum).

See bibliography at the end of Chapter 1.

Fig. 2-9. Diagram showing transducer position (A) and echo (B) from plane 1 as described in Figure 2-8. The superior (*SVC*) and inferior (*IVC*) venae cavae are viewed in long axis as they enter the right atrium (*RA*). The right pulmonary artery (*RPA*) is seen in cross section behind the SVC. This is a good view for standardized measurements of the RPA. The most rightward aspect of the interatrial septum lies in front of the left atrium (*LA*), near the entrance of the right pulmonary veins. The right atrial appendage (*RAA*) may be seen rising anteriorly from the RA.

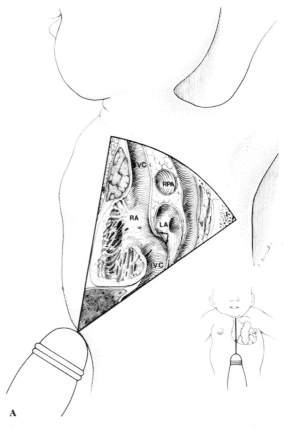

A

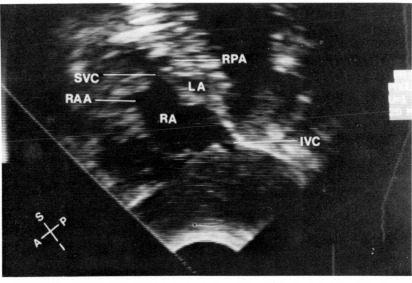

B

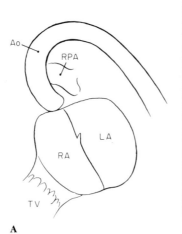

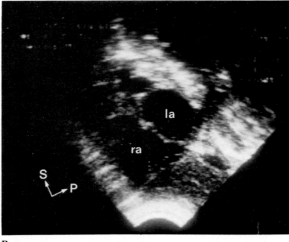

A   B

Fig. 2-10. Diagram (A) and echo (B) of subxiphoid position (S2) crosses the atria at the midpoint of the interatrial septum, the foramen ovale. This plane is orthogonal to the subxiphoid 4- chamber view (L2). A portion of the tricuspid annulus is seen anteriorly. *Ao* = aorta; *LA, la* = left atrium; *RA, ra* = right atrium; *RPA* = right pulmonary artery; *TV* = tricuspid valve.

Fig. 2-11. Diagram (A), cut section of dog heart (B), and echo (C) from subxiphoid (S3) transducer position display the right ventricular (*RV*) inflow and tricuspid orifice. The membranous and inflow areas of the ventricular septum are seen. This plane also displays the aortic annulus, a tangential view of the left ventricular outflow tract, and the proximal portion of the anterior mitral leaflet. A portion of the left atrium (*LA*) is seen posteriorly. *Ao* = aorta; *TV* = tricuspid valve.

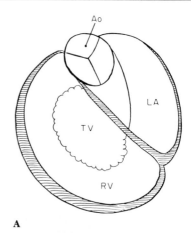

A

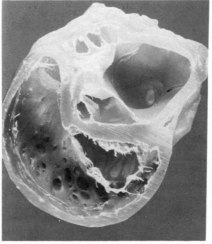

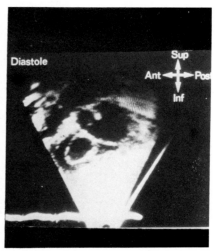

B   C

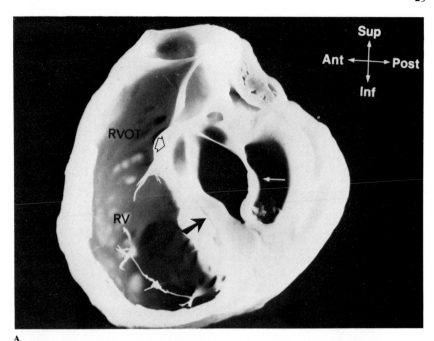

A

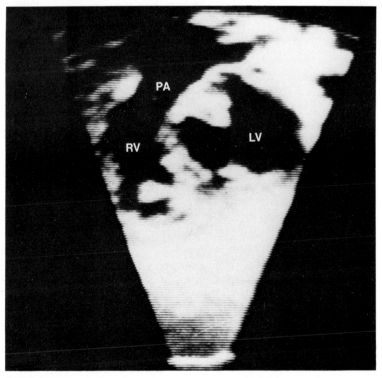

B

Fig. 2-12. Cut section of dog heart (A) and echo (B) of subxiphoid (S4) view, represented by plane 4 in Figure 2-8, are aligned in the long axis of right ventricular outflow tract (*RVOT*). Since the RVOT and left ventricular (LV) outflow tract cross at nearly right angles, this position provides a short-axis view of the LV at the level of the anterior mitral leaflet (*solid white arrow*). This view, similar to the high transverse parasternal view, is optimal for display of the infundibular septum (*open arrow*) and lower trabecular septum (*black arrow*). *PA* = pulmonary artery; *RV* = right ventricle.

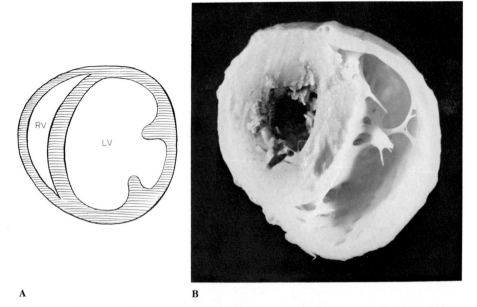

A

B

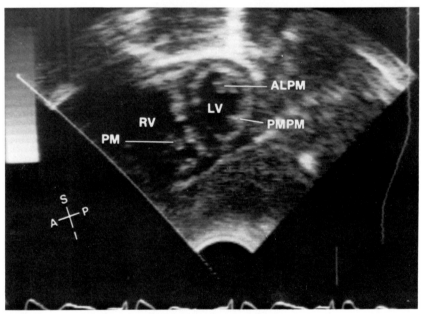

C

Fig. 2-13. Diagram (A), cut section of dog heart (B), and echo (C) of short axis of left ventricle (*LV*) as seen in subxiphoid (S5) view. This plane crosses the LV at the level of the papillary muscles (*PM*), seen protruding into the LV cavity. The midmuscular portion of the interventricular septum is displayed between the right ventricular (*RV*) and LV cavities. The transducer may be swept further leftward (not shown) to display the LV apex and apical portion of the interventricular septum. *ALPM* = anterolateral papillary muscle; *PMPM* = posterior-medial papillary muscle.

CHAPTER 3

Suprasternal Approach

SUPRASTERNAL
NOTCH VIEWS

With the shoulders supported by a pillow, the head falls back in the cooper-ative or unconscious patient so that the transducer can be directed from the suprasternal notch (SSN) or right supraclavicular area and aligned either parallel or perpendicular to the transverse aorta. The left aortic arch may be more easily displayed from the right base of the neck (supraclavicular area) and the right aortic arch from the left base of the neck because the arches are placed at an advantageous distance from the transducer.

From the SSN, the echo beam can be directed into a nearly coronal or parasagittal plane (relative to the trunk), much like the subxiphoid views (Fig. 3-1). With some rotation, the parasagittal view displays the long axis of the aortic arch and the short axis of the right pulmonary artery (RPA) (Fig. 3-2). The coronal view displays the length of RPA and a tangential view of the ascending aorta and arch (Fig. 3-3). The SSN approach provides an ex-cellent view of venous anatomy in the upper mediastinum and is very useful in defining pulmonary venous connections.

See bibliography at the end of Chapter 1.

Fig. 3-1. Drawing displays the trans-ducer position for display of the aortic arch from the suprasternal notch and subxiphoid transducer positions.

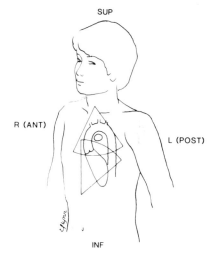

27

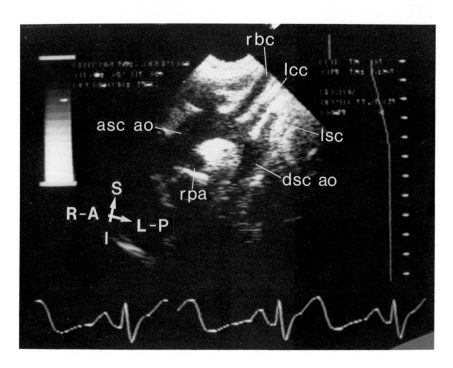

Fig. 3-2. Suprasternal notch view of the long axis of a left aortic arch. This view is almost identical to the high right sternal border and intermediate subxiphoid views. The right pulmonary artery (*rpa*) is seen in cross section. This is a standard view for measurement of RPA size. *asc ao* = ascending aorta; *dsc ao* = descending aorta; *lcc* = left common carotid artery; *lsc* = left subclavian artery; *rbc* = right brachiocephalic artery.

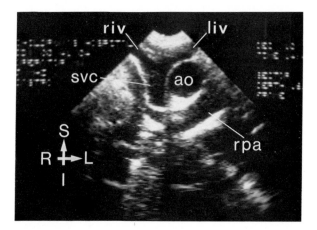

Fig. 3-3. Suprasternal notch short-axis view of aorta (*ao*) displays the long axis of the right pulmonary artery (*rpa*). This echo plane is similar to the subxiphoid long-axis view. *liv* = left innominate vein; *riv* = right innominate vein; *svc* = superior vena cava.

Interrelationships of Different Views

The multiplicity of transducer positions utilized in the complete echocardiographic examination may seem complex and confusing when first encountered, but may be simplified to three basic planes (Fig. 4-1).

LEFT VENTRICULAR OUTFLOW LONG AXIS

The parasternal long-axis, apical 2-chamber, and subxiphoid long-axis (L3) views all display the aorta-to-apex length of the left ventricle (LV). The parasternal and apical 2-chamber views display the anteroposterior (A-P) coordinates of the LV; therefore, these views demonstrate the subaortic, midmuscular, and apical portions of the interventricular septum and the posterior LV free wall (Fig. 4-2).

The subxiphoid long-axis view of the LV outflow tract is at right angles to the parasternal long-axis and apical 2-chamber views. The subxiphoid view displays the right-left coordinates of the LV outflow tract. The membranous interventricular septum, a rightward structure, is displayed from this view. The lateral LV free wall is displayed from this view (see Fig. 2-6A, B).

Fig. 4-1. Drawing displays the three simplified planes utilized by echocardiography to display all cardiac structures. The LV long-axis, short-axis, and 4-chamber views are mutually orthogonal planes, allowing cardiac structures to be represented by anteroposterior, superoinferior, and right-left coordinates.

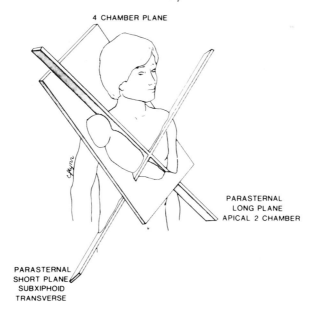

4 CHAMBER PLANE

PARASTERNAL
LONG PLANE
APICAL 2 CHAMBER

PARASTERNAL
SHORT PLANE
SUBXIPHOID
TRANSVERSE

PARASTERNAL
LONG AXIS

COORDINATES: A–P, Sup (R) – Inf (L)

SEGMENTS VIEWED: Midmuscular and Outflow
Septum, Posterior Free Wall

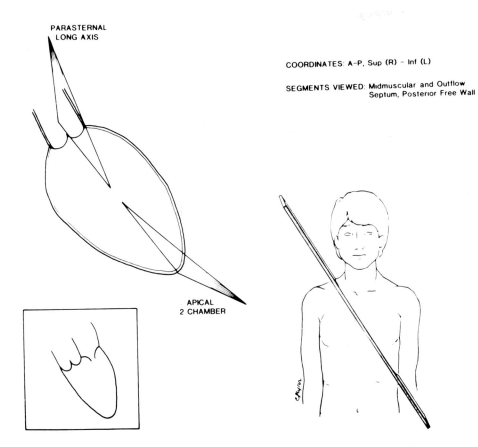

APICAL
2 CHAMBER

Fig. 4-2. Diagram shows plane of transducer beam, transducer positions, and representative slice of the parasternal long-axis and apical 2-chamber view.

PART I. Imaging the Normal Heart

LEFT VENTRICULAR
INFLOW LONG AXIS

The apical and subxiphoid (L2) 4-chamber views demonstrate the midportion of the interatrial septum, the crux of heart, the atrioventricular (A-V) valves, and the lengths of the inflow septum and lateral free walls (Fig. 4-3). The exact inclination of the apical 4-chamber plane varies according to the size and position of the heart. Limited sweeping of the transducer is possible from this position. From both apical and subxiphoid positions, one must sweep the transducer posteriorly in order to demonstrate structures such as the posterior muscular septum and coronary sinus.

Fig. 4-3. Diagram shows plane and transducer positions of apical and subxiphoid 4-chamber views.

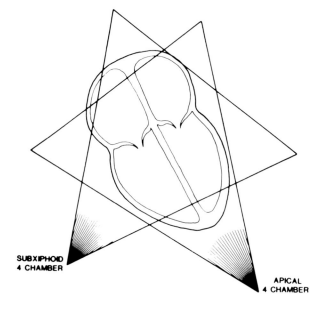

COORDINATES: R–L, Sup–Inf

SEGMENTS VIEWED: Inflow Septum (Mem, AVC, Musc), Lateral Free Wall

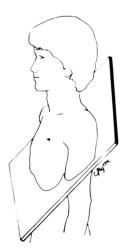

SUBXIPHOID
4 CHAMBER

APICAL
4 CHAMBER

CHAPTER 4. Interrelationships of Different Views

LEFT VENTRICULAR SHORT AXIS

The parasternal and subxiphoid short-axis sweeps provide similar serial cross sections of LV outflow from base to apex (Fig. 4-4). As the long axes of the right ventricle (RV) and LV are nearly perpendicular, a view of the LV short axis displays the RV long axis. The parasternal and subxiphoid short-axis views differ slightly in angulation and in the adequacy of the acoustic window. The parasternal view affords a superior image of the pulmonary artery bifurcation, and the subxiphoid view better displays the subpulmonary area from RV apex to pulmonary valve. These two transducer positions provide similar equatorial short-axis images of the LV for volume or area measurements.

Fig. 4-4. Diagram shows plane of transducer beam, transducer positions, and representative slice of the parasternal and subxiphoid short-axis views as well as direction of sweep from base to apex.

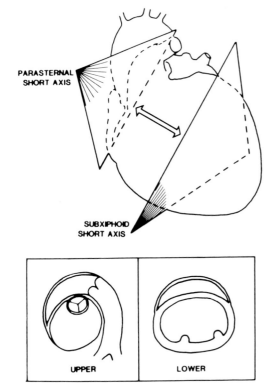

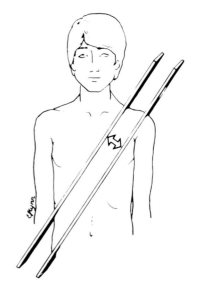

COORDINATES: A–P, R (Inf) – L (Sup)

SEGMENTS VIEWED: Inflow Septum (AVC, Mem, Musc),
Infundibular Septum,
Lateral and Posterior Free Wall

PARASTERNAL SHORT AXIS

SUBXIPHOID SHORT AXIS

UPPER   LOWER

PART I. Imaging the Normal Heart

The long axes of LV inflow and outflow tracts form an acute angle, whereas the long axes of RV inflow and outflow tracts form a much wider, almost 90° angle. The long axis of RV inflow is displayed from the apical 4-chamber view. The subxiphoid 4-chamber view displays only a portion of the RV inflow tract because the beam encounters the right heart from a more posterior position and the RV is a more anterior structure. The long axis of RV outflow tract is displayed from oblique transverse parasternal and subxiphoid short-axis (S4) views of the LV. Since the long axes of the RV and LV outflow tracts are nearly perpendicular, the RV long-axis view and the LV short-axis view are almost identical.

In the preceding chapters, an organized method for imaging the normal heart has been described and provides a general orientation of the heart and great vessels. Many normal structures, like the aortic arch, are variable in position. In complex heart disease, the positions of cardiac structures are so altered that they are best displayed from nonstandard transducer positions. Nevertheless, the technique of sweeping the beam from cardiac base to apex and in the orthogonal plane has proved to be consistently useful in identifying the spatial positions of all cardiac structures and defining their base relationships. Specific anatomic features are defined by rotating or angling the transducer until the structure in question is displayed to best advantage.

See bibliography at the end of Chapter 1.

Shunt Lesions

Atrial Septal Defect

ANATOMY

Secundum-type atrial septal defects (ASDs) result from a deficiency of the septum primum, the flap valve of the foramen ovale. Occupying a central portion of the interatrial septum, the defect is bordered superiorly by the superior limbic band and extends a variable distance inferiorly and posteriorly (Fig. 5-1). The defect may be round, slit-shaped, or formed by multiple fenestrations. A patent foramen ovale is an interatrial communication in the same location, caused not by deficiency of the septum primum, but by the failure of the septum primum to seal against the "door jamb" of the limbus. The foramen ovale is often stretched, with a redundant septum primum billowing into the right or left atrium (RA and LA, respectively), according to the relative interatrial pressures. From patient to patient, there is great variation in size of the foramen ovale and the amount of septum primum covering it.

Primum-type ASDs occur in the leftward portion of the interatrial septum, immediately above the atrioventricular (A-V) valves, and are almost always associated with a cleft anterior mitral leaflet.

Sinus venosus–type ASDs are found at the most rightward extent of the interatrial septum and may be located superiorly, near the orifice of the superior vena cava (SVC), or inferiorly, near the orifice of the inferior vena cava (IVC). Both types of defects may be associated with anomalies of pulmonary venous return.

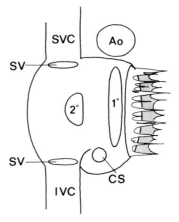

Fig. 5-1. Diagram shows position of interatrial septal defects. The secundum defect (*2°*) is centrally placed at the fossa ovalis. The primum defect (*1°*) lies to the left of the fossa ovalis. The primum defect is usually elliptic, extending superiorly toward the aorta (*Ao*) and inferiorly toward the coronary sinus (*CS*). The rightward-placed sinus venosus defects (*SV*) may be positioned near the orifice of the superior vena cava (*SVC*) or inferior vena cava (*IVC*).

Coronary sinus ASDs are found in the roof of the coronary sinus. The resulting left-to-right interatrial shunt results in dilatation of the coronary sinus as well as the right heart structures.

DIAGNOSTIC ECHO
FINDINGS

A secundum ASD appears as an absence or deficiency of septum primum in the region of the foramen ovale. In contrast, when there is a patent foramen ovale, there is an adequate, or even a redundant, septal primum that is not continuous with the upper margin of the foramen.

A primum ASD is represented by dropout of the leftward margin of the atrial septum, immediately above the A-V valve annulus. Larger defects may be continuous with secundum defects, in which case there is virtual absence of an atrial septum except for a single band crossing the atria. A cleft mitral valve (trileaflet left A-V valve) attached to the crest of the interventricular septum (IVS) is almost invariably associated with a primum ASD.

Sinus venosus defects appear as dropout in the interatrial septum immediately adjacent to the junction with the SVC or IVC. In the more common superiorly placed defects, there is a deficiency in the wall between the SVC junction and the right pulmonary veins (RPVs). When the upper RPV drains to the SVC, this connection may be visualized from views that image the right caval border (subxiphoid, right parasternal, or suprasternal notch [SSN] views). Inferiorly placed sinus venosus defects are immediately to the right of the coronary ostium at the mouth of the IVC.

INDIRECT FINDINGS

Right heart dilation is present when there is significant left-to-right shunting at the atrial level. The convexity of the IVS bulges toward the left ventricle (LV) during diastole when there is a significant right ventricular (RV) volume overload.

EXAMINATION
TECHNIQUE

The technical challenges of visualizing ASDs are (1) imaging the weakly reflective septum primum, (2) scanning all portions of the interatrial septum and coronary sinus, and (3) visualizing all defects in more than one plane.

The septum primum is a thin membrane that may bulge into the RA or LA (Fig. 5-2A to C). Therefore, the membrane is more easily imaged when the ultrasound beam is perpendicular, or nearly so, to the interatrial septum (Fig. 5-2A). The subxiphoid and right sternal border approaches are most nearly perpendicular to the interatrial septum.

CHAPTER 5. Atrial Septal Defect

The interatrial septum must be scanned vertically from its extreme right border to its left margin at the A-V junction and horizontally from its inferior margin at the entrance of the IVC to its superior margin at the junction with the SVC (Fig. 5-3). The subxiphoid position provides the best acoustic window for sweeping because the transducer can be rotated through a wide area without losing skin contact. In large patients, the superior borders of the atria may not be within the focal range of available transducers: Limited scanning can be achieved by sliding the transducer up and down the right sternal border in parasagittal and transverse planes. This must be performed with the patient in a steep right-lateral decubitus position.

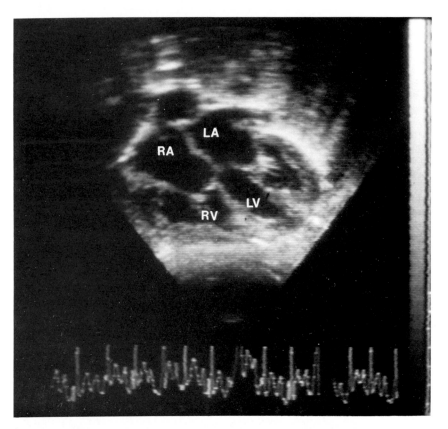

A

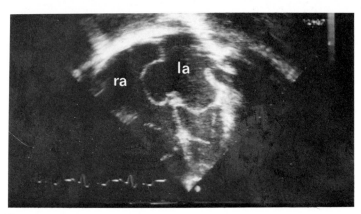

B

Fig. 5-2. (A) Four-chamber or midatrial long-axis subxiphoid view of foramen ovale. In this patient, the position of the interatrial septum is neutral. (B) A redundant septum primum bulges into the right atrium in this patient with a restrictive cardiomyopathy. (C) A redundant septum primum bulges leftward in this patient with pulmonary atresia and intact ventricular septum. *LA, la* = left atrium; *LV, lv* = left ventricle; *RA, ra* = right atrium; *RV, rv* = right ventricle.

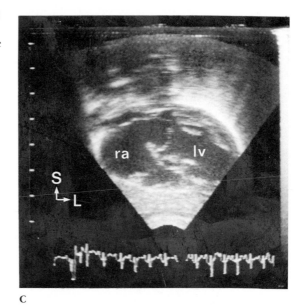

C

Fig. 5-3. Heart viewed from the right side. Positions of the horizontal scan plane from subxiphoid long-axis views, seen on edge, are indicated by lines (*1*) and (*2*). The atria are scanned from inferior (*IVC*) to superior vena cava (*SVC*). The atria must also be vertically scanned in short axis (see Chap. 2). *Ao* = aorta.

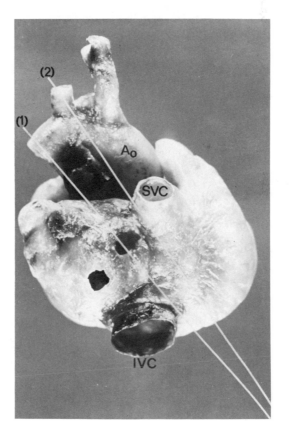

CHAPTER 5. Atrial Septal Defect

An interatrial defect may be elliptic, therefore, the size is better assessed when viewed in orthogonal planes. Viewing in multiple planes also guards against misinterpretation of artifactual dropout.

Secundum atrial defects are best visualized from midatrial views in both long- and short-axis subxiphoid planes (Fig. 5-4A to C) (see Chap. 3).

Fig. 5-4. (A) Subxiphoid long-axis view of large secundum defect. Note normal relation of right upper pulmonary vein (*arrow*) to the superior rim of foramen ovale. (B) Subxiphoid short-axis view of medium-sized secundum defect (*arrow*). (C) Subxiphoid short-axis view of large secundum defect. Note the rim of superior limbic band (*arrow*) that separates the superior vena cava (*SVC*) from the margin of the defect. The presence of this remnant of septum distinguishes a large secundum defect from a sinus venosus–type defect. *LA* = left atrium; *RA* = right atrium.

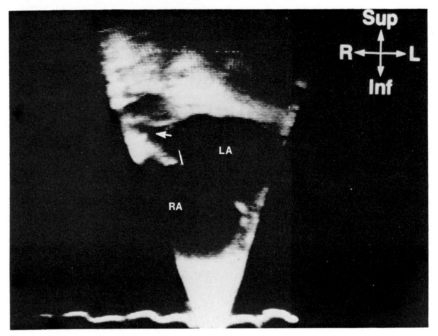

A

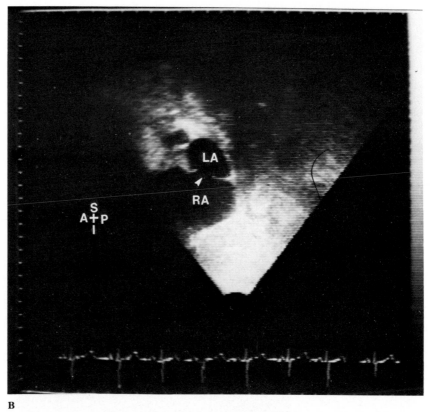

B

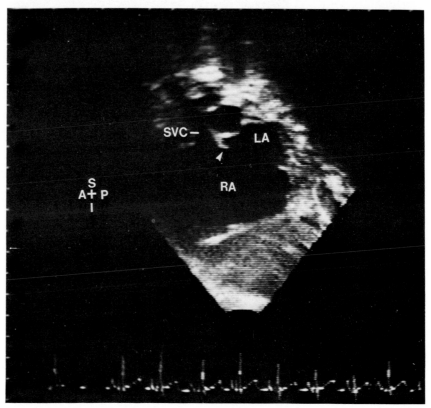

C

Most primum-type atrial defects are easily visualized from the precordial, apical, and subxiphoid positions because this portion of the interatrial septum is thick and straight and there is no confusion with artifactual dropout (Fig. 5-5A to C). The apical and subxiphoid 4-chamber views best demonstrate the relationship between the atrial defect, A-V valves, and the IVS. Rarely, the interatrial communication in complete A-V canal (A-V septal) defect is quite small and limited to an area near the aortic root. In such cases, the transducer must be swept superiorly from a 4-chamber view in order to recognize these small defects. The subxiphoid long-axis view of LV outflow exhibits the goose-neck deformity of the LV outflow in a similar fashion to a right anterior oblique LV angiogram (Fig. 5-6A, B). The subxiphoid and the parasternal short-axis views of the LV show the superior and inferior components of the left A-V valve (cleft anterior mitral leaflet) attached to the midportion of the IVS (Fig. 5-6C, D, E).

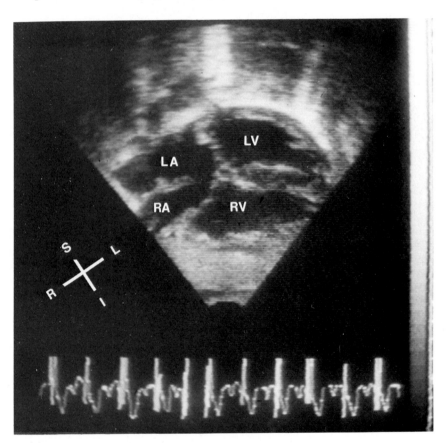

A

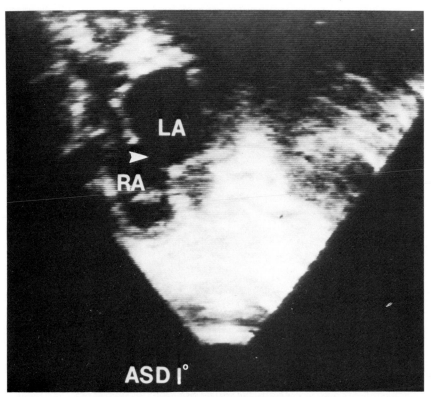

B

Fig. 5-5. (A) Primum atrial septal defect (*ASD 1°*) viewed from subxiphoid 4-chamber view. The defect is at the left margin of the atrial septum, immediately adjacent to the atrioventricular valves. (B) Short-axis subxiphoid view of ASD 1° (*arrow*) was obtained by angling the transducer slightly to the left of the midatrium (area of the foramen ovale). This view is difficult to interpret, unless viewed as a part of a scan, because of the absence of specific landmarks. (C) Apical 4-chamber view in a patient with ASD 1°. *LA, la* = left atrium; *LV, lv* = left ventricle; *RA, ra* = right atrium; *RV, rv* = right ventricle.

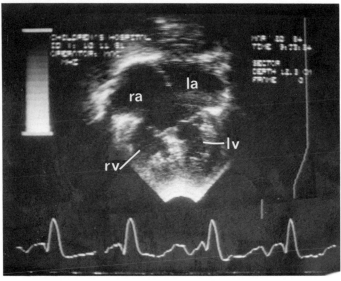

C

CHAPTER 5. Atrial Septal Defect

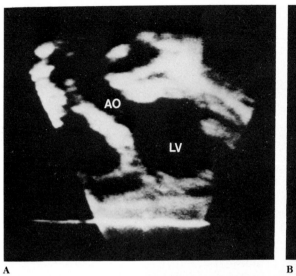

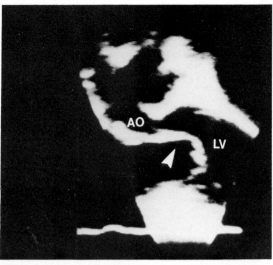

A B

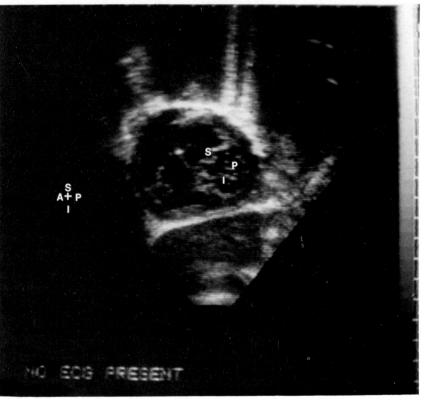

C

PART II. Shunt Lesions

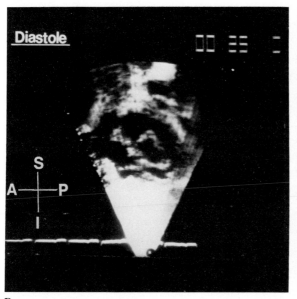

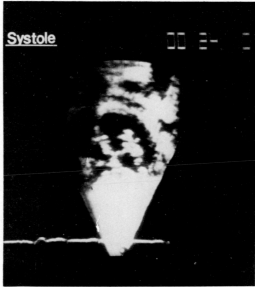

D

E

Fig. 5-6. Subxiphoid long-axis view of left ventricular outflow (L3) in a normal patient (A) and a patient with atrioventricular septal (atrioventricular canal) defect (B). Note that in B the medial border of the left ventricle (*LV*) is formed by the atrioventricular valve (*arrow*), resulting in the goose-neck deformity. Subxiphoid short-axis (S4) view of mid-LV (C) demonstrates the trileaflet nature of the left atrio-ventricular valve. The superior (*S*) and inferior (*I*) leaflets of left atrioventricular valve are attached to the crest of the interventricular septum. The posterior leaflet (*P*) is normal in position. Cleft mitral valve viewed from subxiphoid short-axis (S4) plane shows position of trileaflet mitral valve in diastole (D) and systole (E) as the valve appears to open toward the interventricular septum. *AO* = aorta.

CHAPTER 5. Atrial Septal Defect

The superiorly located sinus venosus ASD is displayed from the subxiphoid approach by extreme rightward short-axis or superiorly directed long-axis views. Either view intersects the junction between rightward and superior portion of the interatrial septum and the SVC (Fig. 5-7A, B). The long-axis view also demonstrates the position of the RPVs relative to the interatrial septum. This is important because of the common association of partial anomalous pulmonary venous return with this type of defect.

The IVC-type of sinus venosus defect is best seen from subxiphoid long- and short-axis views displaying the lower rightward portions of the interatrial septum (inferior limbic band) just above the entrance of the IVC to the RA (Fig. 5-8).

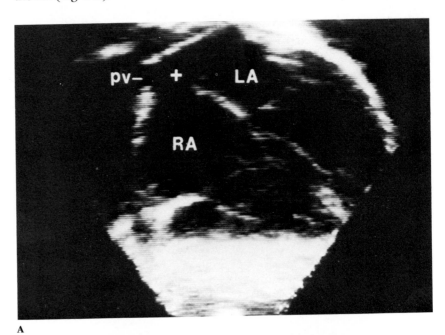

A

Fig. 5-7. (A) Subxiphoid long-axis view of superiorly placed sinus venosus defect was obtained by sweeping superiorly from the 4-chamber view. Note how the right upper pulmonary vein (*pv*) enters the atrial cavity at the site of the defect (+). (B) Companion extreme rightward subxiphoid short-axis view. Sinus venosus defect is represented by dropout of the interatrial septum adjacent to the opening of the superior vena cava (*svc*). Note the absence of superior limbic band between svc and defect compared to Figure 5-4C. *LA, la* = left atrium; *RA, ra* = right atrium.

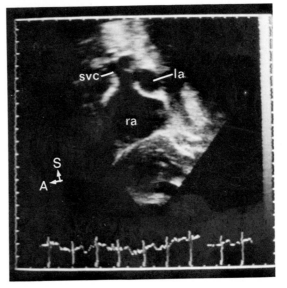

B

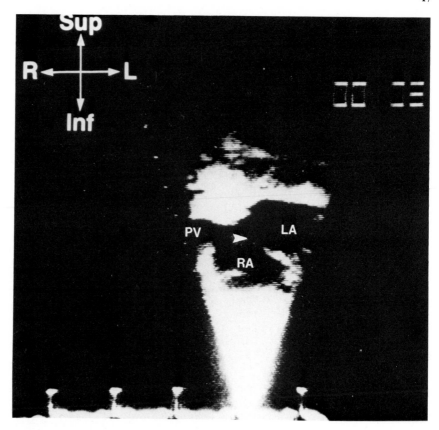

Fig. 5-8. Low subxiphoid long-axis view (L1) of patient with inferior type of sinus venosus atrial septal defect (*arrow*). Note ambiguous position of lower right pulmonary vein (*PV*) relative to interatrial septum. Eustachian valve must be separately identified in order to avoid confusing it with the rim of interatrial septum visualized here between the right (*RA*) and left (*LA*) atria.

CHAPTER 5. Atrial Septal Defect

Sinus septal defects may be visualized in the roof of a large coronary sinus. The coronary sinus should be examined in long axis from posteriorly angled apical and subxiphoid 4-chamber views, as well as in short-axis subxiphoid sweeps (Fig. 5-9A, B) from coronary sinus mouth to tail.

Forceful injection of dextrose or electrolyte solution, blood, or indocyanine green dye into the systemic vein fills the right heart with echo-dense contrast material. When this contrast effect fills the RA with dense bubbles, unopacified blood from a left-to-right atrial shunt will create a negative contrast effect in the area of the defect, which extends into the RA for a variable distance. In some patients, a small amount of contrast passes from the RA to LA despite a predominant left-to-right shunt. This effect is accentuated by the Valsalva maneuver.

Fig. 5-9. (A) Subxiphoid short-axis view demonstrates a left superior vena cava (*l-svc*) to coronary sinus (*cs*) in a patient with an intact CS septum. (B) Similar subxiphoid short-axis view in a patient with a sinus septal defect in the roof of CS. *la* = left atrium; *ra* = right atrium.

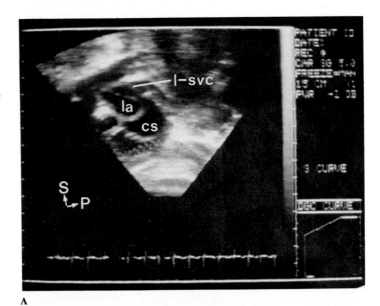

A

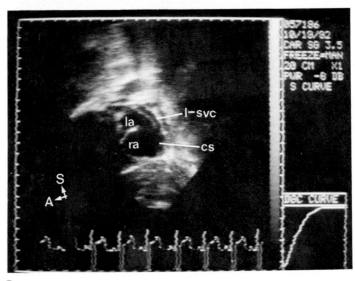

B

PART II. Shunt Lesions

False-positive diagnosis of secundum atrial defect may arise from artifactual dropout of the fossa ovalis when the atrial septum is imaged from only the left parasternal and apical positions. This problem can be avoided by confirming the presence of dropout from the subxiphoid or right sternal border view. Another source of false-positive diagnosis is the misidentification of the mouth of a dilated coronary sinus as an inferiorly located sinus venosus or primum ASD (Fig. 5-10). Familiarity with the position of the coronary ostium will prevent this error. Additionally, the body of the coronary sinus will be seen extending posteriorly from a dilated ostium, along the left A-V groove.

False-negative diagnosis of ASD is most often caused by inadequate scanning due to body habitus or unfamiliarity with some areas of the atrial septum. The inferior rightward portion of the interatrial septum, site of the inferior type of sinus venosus defect, is infrequently scanned in many laboratories, resulting in a false-negative diagnosis of this uncommon anomaly. Defects in the roof of the coronary sinus are also frequently overlooked as a source of interatrial shunting.

Fig. 5-10. Low subxiphoid 4-chamber view shows dilated coronary sinus (*CS*). The mouth of the CS appears as a gap at the lower margin of the interatrial septum, but visualization of the body of the CS lying beneath the left atrium (*LA*) and awareness of inferior transducer position should prevent confusion. *RA* = right atrium.

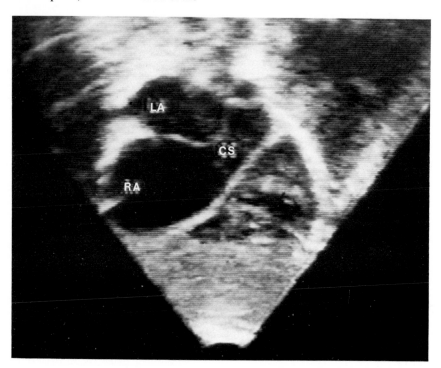

Rarely, multiple small perforations within the flap valve of the foramen ovale (septum primum) are too small to visualize, yet they allow a significant left-to-right shunt. Contrast injection should identify the location of the defect(s).

The size of the RV should always be assessed when entertaining the diagnosis of ASD. An RV of normal size in the presence of an apparent interatrial communication should raise a suspicion of false-positive diagnosis. Conversely, a dilated RV in the presence of an apparently intact interatrial septum should provide incentive to continue the search for a defect or anomalous pulmonary venous connection (see Chap. 9).

BIBLIOGRAPHY

Beppu, S., Nimura, Y., Sakakibara, H., et al. Mitral cleft in ostium primum atrial septal defect assessed by cross-sectional echocardiography. *Circulation* 62:1099, 1980.

Bierman, F. Z., and Williams, R. W. Subxiphoid two-dimensional imaging of the interatrial septum in infants and neonates with congenital heart defects. *Circulation* 60:80, 1979.

Casta, A., Casta, D., Sapir, D. W., et al. True congenital aneurysm of the septum primum not associated with obstructive right-or-left-sided lesions: Identified by two-dimensional echocardiography and angiography in a newborn. *Pediatr. Cardiol.* 4:159, 1983.

Cohen, B. E., Winer, H. E., and Kronzon, I. Echocardiographic findings in patients with left superior vena cava and dilated coronary sinus. *Am. J. Cardiol.* 44:158, 1979.

Freedom, R. M., Culham, J. A. G., and Rowe, R. D. Left atrial to coronary sinus fenestration (partially unroofed coronary sinus): Morphological and angiographic observations. *Br. Heart J.* 46:63, 1981.

Gondi, B., and Nanda, N. C. Two-dimensional echocardiographic features of atrial septal aneurysms. *Circulation* 63:452, 1981.

Iliceto, S., Antonelli, G., Sorino, M., et al. Detection of atrial septal defect of right sternal border echocardiography. *Am. J. Cardiol.* 54:376, 1984.

Kronik, G., Slany, J., and Moesslacher, H. Contrast m-mode echocardiography in the diagnosis of atrial septal defects in acyanotic patients. *Circulation* 59:372, 1979.

Lieppe, W., Seallion, R., Behar, V. S., et al. Two-dimensional echocardiographic findings in atrial septal defect. *Circulation* 56:447, 1977.

Nasser, F. N., Tajik, A. J., Seward, J. B., et al. Diagnosis of sinus venosus atrial septal defect by two-dimensional echocardiography. *Mayo Clin. Proc.* 56:568, 1981.

Rose, A. G., Beckman, C. B., and Edwards, J. E. Communication between coronary sinus and left atrium. *Br. Heart J.* 36:182, 1974.

Sahn, D. J., Allen, H. D., Anderson, R., et al. Echocardiographic diagnosis of atrial septal aneurysm in an infant with hypoplastic right heart syndrome. *Chest* 73:227, 1978.

Shub, C., Dimopoulos, I. N., Seward, J. B., et al. Sensitivity of two-dimensional echocardiography in the direct visualization of atrial septal defect utilizing the subcostal approach: Experience with 154 patients. *J. Am. Coll. Cardiol.* 2:127, 1983.

Tei, C., Tanaka, H., Kashima, T., et al. Real-time cross-sectional echocardiographic evaluation of the interatrial septum by right atrium—interatrial septum—left atrium direction of ultrasound beam. *Circulation* 60:539, 1979.

Yeager, H., Chin, A. J., and Sanders, S. B. Subxiphoid two-dimensional echocardiographic diagnosis of coronary sinus septal defects. *Am. J. Cardiol.* 54:686, 1984.

Yoshida, H., Funabashi, T., Nakaya, S., et al. Sub-xiphoid cross-sectional echocardiographic imaging of the "goose-neck" deformity in endocardial cushion defect. *Circulation* 62:1319, 1980.

Ventricular Septal Defect

ANATOMY

The interventricular septum (IVS) is a complex, curved structure, consisting of a smooth component close to the atrioventricular (A-V) valves, a heavily trabeculated lower muscular component, and a smooth infundibular, or outflow, component that separates the subaortic and subpulmonary outflow areas. Ventricular septal defects (VSDs) may be categorized into five major types (Fig. 6-1).

Perimembranous defects (also known as subaortic or conoventricular defects) are located at the junction between the annuli of the aortic and tricuspid valves. These defects are usually small and oval-shaped when located entirely within the membranous septum, but are larger when extending into other parts of the septum. A complete or partial fibrous rim enhances the echocardiographic appearance of perimembranous defects by acting as a specular reflector. Accessory tissue related to the tricuspid valve may overlie and partially obscure these defects, forming an aneurysm of the membranous septum. Perimembranous defects are usually isolated but may be associated with other VSDs.

A VSD *of the A-V canal type (inlet defect)* lies behind the septal tricuspid leaflet and extends to the A-V valve annulus. In complete A-V septal defects, the A-V valve leaflet forms the upper border of the interventricular portion of the defect. This type of defect may occur as an isolated lesion, but is commonly a component of a complete A-V septal defect (see Chap. 7).

An *anterior malalignment type of defect* (also known as subaortic outflow defect) is often associated with conotruncal defects such as tetralogy of Fallot, double outlet right ventricle (DORV), and transposition of the great arteries. This defect is created by inferior and leftward displacement of the infundibular septum (also known as crista supraventricularis or outflow septum), leaving a space between the lower margin of this structure and the trabecular muscular septum. It is almost invariably a large defect, lying above the tricuspid valve. There may be variable hypoplasia of the infundibular septum in addition to malalignment. The malalignment defect is easily recognized by echocardiography because it is large and unobscured by other structures.

A *posterior malalignment defect* is caused by abnormal posterior location of the outflow septum into the left ventricular (LV) outflow tract. The outflow tract may be narrowed by the position of the outflow septum. This lesion is often associated with downstream obstruction of the posterior great artery such as interruption of the aortic arch and coarctation of the aorta.

Subpulmonary, or intracristal, defects are located within the infundibular septum. With normally related great arteries, this defect lies to the left of the subaortic area, extends to the pulmonary annulus, and has an upper fibrous

Fig. 6-1. Heart specimen with right ventricular free wall removed to expose interventricular septal locations of various ventricular septal defects. Perimembranous defects (*1*) lie at the right superior margin of the tricuspid valve. Atrioventricular canal (septal) defects (*2*) lie beneath the septal leaflet of the tricuspid valve and extend to the tricuspid annulus. Malalignment (e.g., conoseptal, subaortic outflow) defects (*3*) lie superior to the attachment of the septal tricuspid leaflet to the papillary muscle of the conus (*arrow*). Subpulmonary defects (*4*) are to the left of malalignment defects and extend to pulmonary annulus. Muscular defects lie within the trabecular septum and may be positioned in the anterior (*5*), middle (*6*), or posterior (*7*) muscular septum.

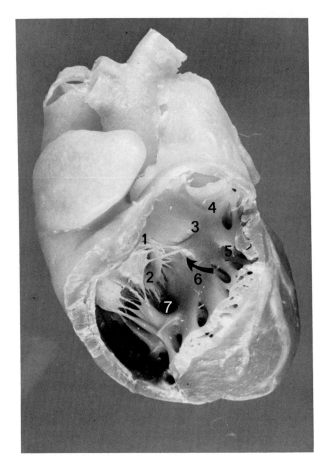

margin. The defect has an intimate relationship to the right coronary cusp of the aortic valve, which may protrude into the opening and obscure it. This phenomenon may result in aortic regurgitation or subpulmonary obstruction.

Muscular defects may lie centrally, posteriorly, inferiorly near the ventricular apex, or anterior to the septal band. These defects have an entirely muscular rim and vary greatly in size and shape. They may be round and unobscured, overlaid by trabeculations, or take the form of tortuous channels. Muscular defects may be associated with other VSDs. In the most extreme form of multiple muscular VSDs, the Swiss-cheese septum, the left septal surface is virtually absent and the right ventricular (RV) trabeculations form the entire septum.

DIAGNOSTIC ECHO FINDINGS

Perimembranous defects are represented by septal dropout in the area behind the septal leaflet of the tricuspid valve and inferior to the rightward border of the aortic annulus. A portion of the septal tricuspid leaflet or accessory A-V valve tissue often overlies the defect. Thus, the defect is more clearly seen in systole, when the A-V valve moves away. The fibrous margin of the defect often creates a specular reflection.

An isolated A-V canal type of VSD, also known as inlet VSD, extends from the fibrous annulus of the tricuspid valve into the muscular septum. The defect may lie entirely beneath the septal tricuspid leaflet, but when large, extends beneath the leaflet into the midmuscular septum. Defects associated with complete or partial A-V canal defects are discussed more fully in Chapter 7.

An anterior malalignment type of VSD appears immediately beneath the posterior semilunar valve cusps. The posterior semilunar root overrides the IVS. The defect lies entirely superior to the tricuspid valve. Thus, in contrast to perimembranous defects, no portion of the septal tricuspid leaflet overlies the malalignment VSD unless the defect extends into the inflow septum. This feature is clearly displayed from parasternal long-axis, apical 2-chamber, and subxiphoid long- and short-axis views. The most common example of anteriorly malaligned defects is seen in tetralogy of Fallot.

The posterior malalignment type of VSD is characterized by posterior displacement of the infundibular septum into the LV outflow tract. This VSD may be associated with significant LV outflow tract narrowing between the outflow septum and the mitral valve. Subxiphoid, right and left parasternal, and apical 2-chamber views demonstrate these features.

The subpulmonary defect appears as dropout within the outflow septum, which extends to the pulmonary annulus. One or two of the aortic cusps may protrude through the defect into the RV outflow tract, obscuring the defect.

Muscular (trabecular) defects may appear anywhere in the mid-, anterior, posterior, or apical muscular septum. They may be a single, large defect or multiple, small ones. Multiple small defects, known as Swiss-cheese septum, may be recognized by discontinuity of the left septal surface. Other defects are fistulous, their tortuous routes not imaged in any single plane. Muscular defects have in common an entirely muscular rim.

It is important to point out that large VSDs often extend into two or more regions of the IVS and will demonstrate composite features of the defects described above; for example, a malalignment or subarterial defect may extend beneath the septal tricuspid leaflet.

INDIRECT FINDINGS

Left atrial (LA) and LV enlargements are two common indirect findings.

Contrast injection into a systemic vein may reveal a negative effect from a left-to-right shunt across the ventricular septum. During catheterization or postoperative studies, LA or LV injection may reveal a positive contrast crossing the ventricular septum at the site of the defect.

Systolic fluttering of the tricuspid valve may be seen on M-mode echo in some patients with membranous defects. In subpulmonary defects, marked systolic vibration of the pulmonary cusps may be noted.

The septal tricuspid leaflet may bulge through a large membranous or A-V canal defect into the LV outflow tract during diastole. The appearance of this

CHAPTER 6. Ventricular Septal Defect

leaflet in the LV does not necessarily indicate overriding tricuspid valve, but strongly suggests deficiency of the IVS behind the leaflet.

Prolapse of an aortic cusp through subpulmonary defect is often associated with findings of aortic regurgitation such as diastolic fluttering of the anterior mitral leaflet (M-mode) or turbulence in the LV outflow tract (Doppler).

EXAMINATION
TECHNIQUE

Transducer positions for viewing the various types of VSDs are shown in Figures 6-2 to 6-4. Precordial views tend to display the more leftward portions of the IVS, where the malalignment, subpulmonary, and leftward-placed muscular defects are found (see Fig. 6-2). The more rightward portions of the IVS are usually not well seen from precordial views, particularly when LV dilatation rotates this part of the IVS even more rightward than usual. The multiple subxiphoid views allow inspection of the entire septum and also place the echo beam at right angles to most of the muscular septum. Localization of the defects is achieved by sweeping the septum from right to left in serial transverse planes (see Fig. 6-3). The apical and subxiphoid 4-chamber views display inflow as well as membranous, posterior, and central muscular defects (Fig. 6-4). Apical defects may also be visualized depending on the quality of the near field. The infundibular, or outflow, septum is not easily seen from this view.

Fig. 6-2. Diagram of the interventricular septum, with points of intersection by left parasternal long-axis (and apical 2-chamber) and short-axis scan planes (*lines*). Note that the long-axis plane crosses sites of malalignment (*3*), midmuscular (*6*), and apical (*8*) defects; a short-axis sweep from base of heart to apex traverses the entire septum, except for the more rightward perimembranous (*1*) and atrioventricular canal (*2*) defects, which are often shielded from view by the sternum.

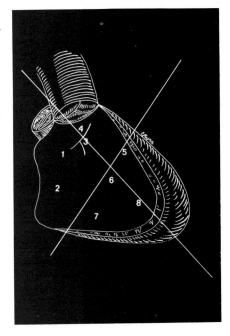

Fig. 6-3. Diagram of the interventricular septum shows subxiphoid
short-axis scan planes (*lines*). Pivoting
transducer from right to left sweeps the
entire septum from atrioventricular
valve annulus to apex.

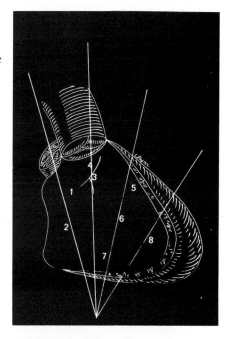

Fig. 6-4. Diagram of the interventricular septum depicts intersection
of apical 4-chamber scan (*lines*). Limited sweeping from the apex covers the
area from the atrioventricular canal (*2*)
and posterior (*7*) defects to perimembranous (*1*), midmuscular (*6*),
and apical defects, but generally does
not reach superiorly to the outflow septal defects. Scan plane of subxiphoid
long-axis views (*not shown*) are
roughly parallel to the lower line
shown here and sweep superiorly to
the pulmonary valve.

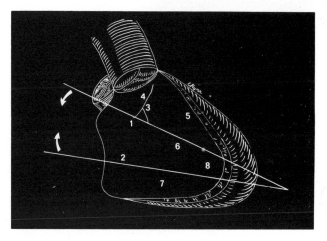

CHAPTER 6. Ventricular Septal Defect

Perimembranous defects are best visualized from short-axis views of the LV obtained from subxiphoid and right and left parasternal transducer positions, but can also be seen from subxiphoid and right parasternal long-axis views, because these planes intersect the rightward border of the LV out-flow tract (Figs. 6-5, 6-6A to C).

A-V septal (inlet) defects are best visualized from apical and subxiphoid 4-chamber views (Fig. 6-7) as well as parasternal, subxiphoid, and right sternal border short-axis views. The malalignment VSD is best imaged from the parasternal and subxiphoid long-axis views, which demonstrate the over-riding great artery, and from the subxiphoid and high transverse parasternal short-axis views, which display the RV outflow tract in long axis (Fig. 6-8A, B). The subpulmonary defect is best demonstrated from subxiphoid (S4) and high left parasternal views angled along the long axis of the RV outflow tract (Fig. 6-9A, B). Both views demonstrate the portion of infundibular (out-flow) septum to the left of the aortic valve.

All portions of the trabecular muscular septum must be intersected in at least two views in order to display the variously placed muscular defects (Fig. 6-10A to C). Ideally, signal amplification and display should be adjusted until the myocardium is faintly seen and the specular echoes are toned down. This adjustment will improve the ability to recognize the margins of a muscular defect and decrease the tendency of specular echoes from a fibrous margin to fill in the defect.

Fig. 6-5. Subxiphoid long-axis view (L3) of left ventricular (*LV*) outflow tract demonstrates perimembranous defect (*arrow*) covered by accessory atrioventricular valve tissue (aneurysm of membranous septum). *AO* = aortic root; *RV* = right ventricle.

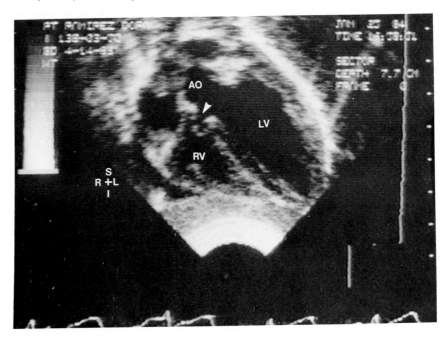

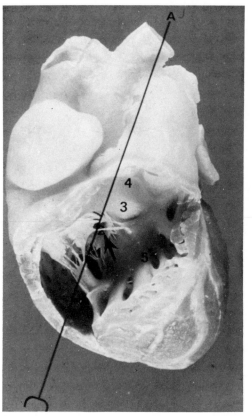

A

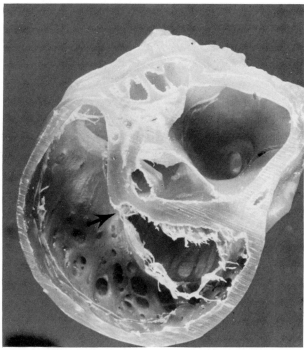

B

Fig. 6-6. (A) Opened right ventricle displays the interventricular septum. Line A indicates the line of intersection of the subxiphoid short-axis plane that demonstrates the perimembranous septum (*arrow*). (B) Cut section of heart corresponds to line A. The region of the perimembranous septum is indicated by the arrow. (C) Subxiphoid short-axis view, corresponding to the plane demonstrated in Figure 6-6B, in a patient with a perimembranous defect (*arrow*). *LV* = left ventricle; *PA* = pulmonary artery; *RV* = right ventricle.

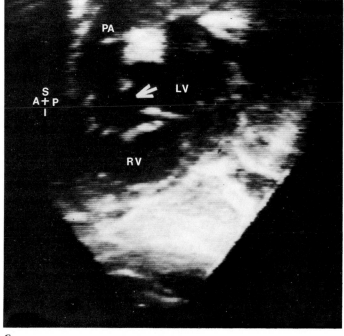

C

CHAPTER 6. Ventricular Septal Defect

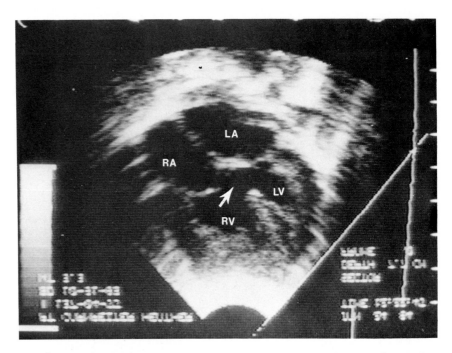

Fig. 6-7. Subxiphoid 4-chamber view of atrioventricular septal (canal) type of isolated ventricular septal defect. Defect (*arrow*) extends superiorly to junction of atrioventricular valve an-

nulus and interatrial septum (crux of heart). *LA* = left atrium; *LV* = left ventricle; *RA* = right atrium; *RV* = right ventricle.

Fig. 6-8. (A) Subxiphoid long-axis view (L3) of left ventricular (*LV*) outflow tract in a patient with tetralogy of Fallot shows aorta (*AO*) straddling the interventricular septum. Note that the defect (*arrows*) lies superior to the tricuspid valve (*TV*). (B) Subxiphoid short-axis view (S3) of malalignment defect in a patient with double outlet right ventricle demonstrates the anteroposterior relationship between the posterior semilunar root, in this case, the pulmonary artery (*PA*), and the lower muscular interventricular septum. The defect lies between the dislocated outflow, or infundibular, septum (*arrow*) and the lower muscular septum. *RV* = right ventricle.

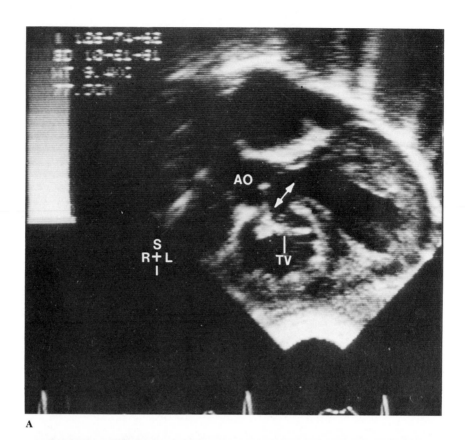

A

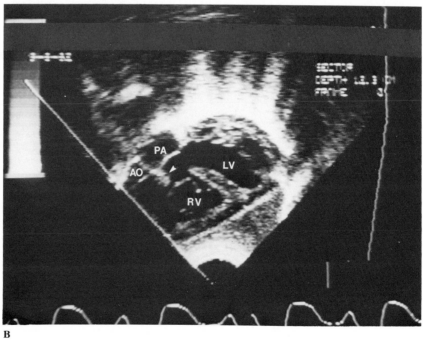

B

CHAPTER 6. Ventricular Septal Defect

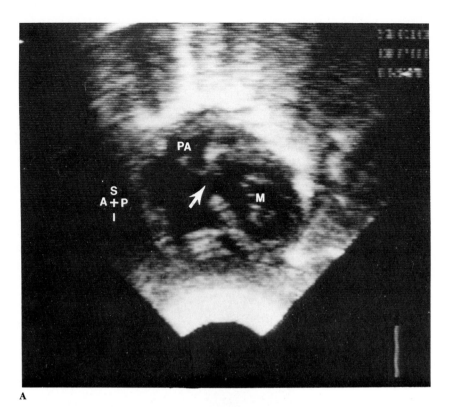

A

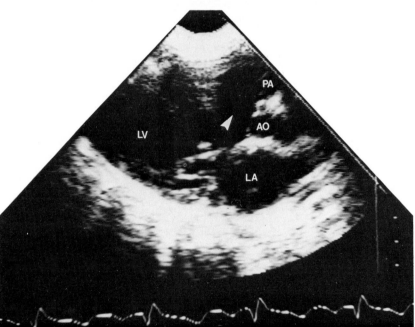

B

Fig. 6-9. Subxiphoid short-axis view (A) and parasternal long-axis view with lateral angulation (B) of subpulmonary ventricular septal defect (*arrows*) extending to pulmonary annulus. Simul- taneous visualization of mitral leaflets (*M*) indicates leftward position of this scan plane. *AO* = aorta; *LA* = left atrium; *LV* = left ventricle; *PA* = pulmonary artery.

PART II. Shunt Lesions

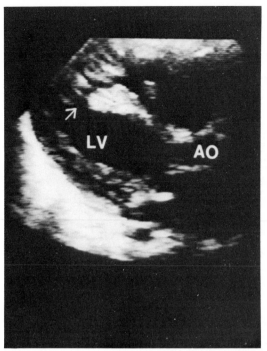

A

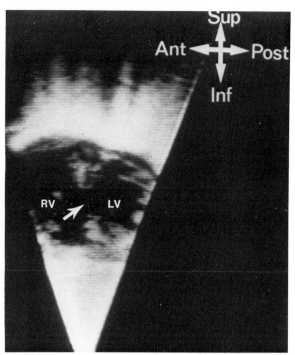

C

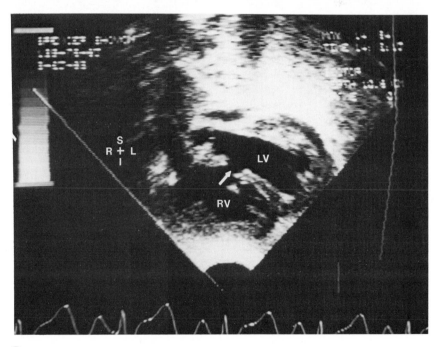

B

Fig. 6-10. Parasternal long-axis view (A) shows small, tortuous muscular ventricular septal defect (*arrow*) lying near apex. Subxiphoid long-axis view (B) of left ventricular (*LV*) outflow tract reveals a moderate-size mid-

muscular septal defect (*arrow*). Subxiphoid short-axis view (C) of LV at level of papillary muscles reveals large, punched-out muscular defect (*arrow*). *AO* = aortic root; *RV* = right ventricle.

CHAPTER 6. Ventricular Septal Defect

PROBLEMS

The tricuspid valve apparatus overlies a portion of the membranous and A-V (canal) septum and may obscure defects in these locations. These defects are best visualized during the beginning of systole, when the tricuspid apparatus moves toward a closed position.

Muscular defects are sometimes difficult to visualize because of a tortuous course or overlying trabeculations. Moreover, they may become smaller during systolic contraction and therefore are better observed during diastole. Likewise, intratrabecular spaces along the right septal surface may mimic a small VSD. The left septal surface must be clearly defined. When discontinuity is observed, the presence of muscular defects should be suspected. Anterior muscular defects are the most difficult to recognize because this part of the septum is usually not scanned as carefully as the central and lower muscular septum.

Herniation of the right aortic cusp through a subpulmonary defect may obscure the interventricular communication.

A large VSD, extending into more than one region of the IVS, cannot be characterized by a single descriptive term. In such cases, it is important to describe all borders of the VSD.

BIBLIOGRAPHY

Bierman, F. Z., Fellows, K., and Williams, R. G. Prospective identification of ventricular septal defects in infancy using subxiphoid two-dimensional echocardiography. *Circulation* 62:807, 1980.

Canale, J. M., Sahn, D. J., Allen, H. D., et al. Factors affecting real-time cross sectional echocardiographic imaging of perimembranous ventricular septal defect. *Circulation* 63:689, 1981.

Capelli, H., Andrade, J. L., and Somerville, J. Classification of the site of ventricular septal defect by 2-dimensional echocardiography. *Am. J. Cardiol.* 51:1474, 1983.

Cheatham, J. P., Latson, L. A., and Gutgesell, H. P. Ventricular septal defect in infancy: Detection by two-dimensional echocardiography. *Am. J. Cardiol.* 47:85, 1981.

Smallhorn, J. F., Anderson, R. H., and MacCartney, F. J. Morphological characterization of ventricular septal defects associated with coarctation of aorta by cross-sectional echocardiography. *Br. Heart J.* 49:485, 1983.

Snider, A. R., Silverman, N. H., Schiller, M. B., and Ports, T. A. Echocardiographic evaluation of ventricular septal aneurysms. *Circulation* 59:920, 1979.

Soto, B., Becker, A. E., Moulaert, A. J., et al. Classification of ventricular septal defects. *Br. Heart J.* 43:332, 1980.

Sutherland, G. R., Godman, M. J., Smallhorn, J. F., et al. Ventricular septal defects: Two-dimensional echocardiographic and morphological correlations. *Br. Heart J.* 47:316, 1982.

Complete Atrioventricular Canal Defects

ANATOMY

Atrioventricular (A-V) canal defects, more recently known as *A-V septal defects*, consist of a central defect with atrial and/or ventricular components. There are no separate A-V valve annuli, but instead a common annulus that straddles the central defect.

The size of the interatrial communication ranges from a large defect, with virtual absence of interatrial septum, to a very small, slitlike defect located just posterior to the aortic root. The ventricular component of the defect is in the A-V septal, or inlet, portion of the interventricular septum (IVS). The size of the ventricular defect ranges from a small space between dense chordal attachments of the A-V valve and the crest of the muscular septum (transitional form of A-V canal defect) to virtual absence of the inlet septum.

The length of the posterior inflow septum is less than the length of the outflow septum in this anomaly. As a result, there is an unusually inferior position of the A-V valves.

The A-V valve deformity involves the entire valve apparatus: annulus, leaflet, chordal attachments, and papillary muscles. A common A-V valve annulus stretches across both ventricles. Occasionally, there is malalignment of the valve with respect to the ventricular septum, resulting in hypoplasia of one of the ventricles. The A-V valves are usually characterized by the morphology and attachments of the superior leaflet(s) (Fig. 7-1A, B). The common A-V valve is variously described as having four to six leaflets. In the Rastelli type A, the superior leaflets do not bridge the ventricular defect and usually attach to the crest of the septum. In the Rastelli-type-C A-V valve, the left superior leaflet bridges the ventricular septal defect (VSD) and may be free floating or have sparse attachments to the crest of the ventricular septum. In the rare Rastelli type B, the bridging leaflets attach to a papillary muscle within the right ventricle (RV). The inferior leaflet is almost always divided and attached to the posterior margin of the VSD. The true posterior leaflet of the left A-V valve is usually normal, but may have decreased width if the papillary muscles of the left ventricles (LVs) are more closely spaced than normal. The tip of the obliquely positioned anterolateral papillary muscle group lies more medially than usual in some patients. In its most extreme form, there is a solitary papillary muscle.

The anatomic features of the A-V valve having the greatest relevance to surgical repair are (1) presence of sufficient tissue for proper coaptation of the leaflets, (2) leaflet mobility (related to density and height of chordal attachments), (3) alignment of the A-V canal over the ventricles, and (4) nature of papillary muscle attachments in the LV.

With some exceptions, the undivided superior leaflet offers enough A-V valve tissue for an adequate repair even if the inferior leaflet is mildly deficient. A divided superior leaflet with dense chordal attachments is more

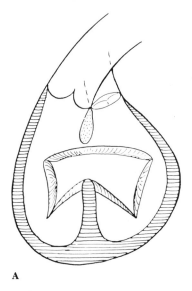 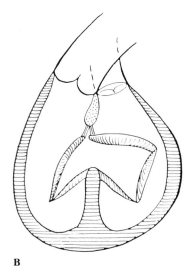

A   B

Fig. 7-1. (A) Typical undivided, or sail, leaflet known as Rastelli type C. The bridging portion of the superior leaflet extends into the right ventricle, bridging the interventricular septum. The bridging leaflet may have sparse medial attachments to the interventricular septum, but often has none. Note that the inferior leaflet typically has medial septal attachments unrelated to superior leaflet morphology. (B) Typical divided superior leaflet with medial chordal attachments to the interventricular septum (Rastelli type A). The inferior leaflet is also attached medially to the interventricular septum.

likely to be incompetent following repair. A mild degree of malalignment of the A-V canal over the ventricles does not present a major surgical problem, particularly when a common superior leaflet allows some flexibility in the placement of the ventricular patch and the apportionment of the A-V valve tissue to RV and LV. Unfortunately, there is at present no quantitative criteria relating the degree of overriding to the surgical outcome.

The tips of the papillary muscles are more closely spaced than usual in a complete A-V canal. The presence of a single LV papillary muscle or very closely spaced papillary muscles may result in a parachute mitral valve deformity if a suture line is placed between the superior and inferior leaflets.

ASSOCIATED LESIONS

Tetralogy of Fallot and double outlet right ventricle (DORV) are uncommon, but troublesome, associated lesions. Minor deviation of the infundibular septum may be difficult to detect when it is separated from the lower muscular septum by a large VSD. Multiple muscular VSDs are occasionally seen, especially in young infants with complete A-V canal defects.

DIAGNOSTIC ECHO FINDINGS

The atrial defect appears as a dropout of echoes from the left-most portion of the interatrial septum, immediately above the A-V valves (Fig. 7-2). If very

PART II. Shunt Lesions

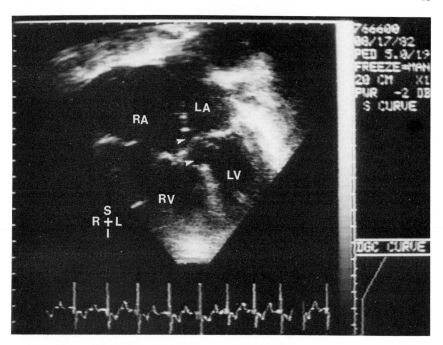

Fig. 7-2. Apical 4-chamber view of complete atrioventricular canal. Atrial defect (*arrow*) and ventricular defect (*arrow*) are seen above and below the atrioventricular valve, respectively. *LA* = left atrium; *LV* = left ventricle; *RA* = right atrium; *RV* = right ventricle.

small, the atrial defect is seen just posterior to the aortic root on superior angulation from the subxiphoid or apical 4-chamber view.

The ventricular defect lies beneath the A-V leaflets. Dense chordal attachments between the leaflet and the crest of the IVS may so completely fill in the space that an interventricular communication cannot be visualized.

The central bridging portion of a sail, or free-floating, superior leaflet appears as a straight line when it opens in diastole, while leaflets with dense, medial chordal attachments do not lie in a straight line in diastole because the central portion is bound down (Fig. 7-3A to C). The distinction between a common bridging leaflet and a divided superior leaflet is more difficult to make. Occasionally, separate right and left portions of the superior leaflet are clearly seen. More commonly, the presence of a divided leaflet is inferred by noting the presence of dense, medial chordal attachments between the leaflet, the IVS, and the resulting configuration in diastole.

The anterolateral papillary muscle of the LV appears in a more medial position than usual, viewed from subxiphoid and parasternal short-axis views. The posterolateral leaflet is shortened when the papillary muscles are more closely spaced. The most extreme form of this phenomenon is shown in Figure 7-4A to F. It is important to recognize that the papillary muscles run obliquely through the ventricle, therefore, there is a discrepancy between echocardiographic studies, which display the body of the papillary muscle, and studies of pathologic specimens, which denote position of papillary muscles at their base.

CHAPTER 7. Complete Atrioventricular Canal Defects

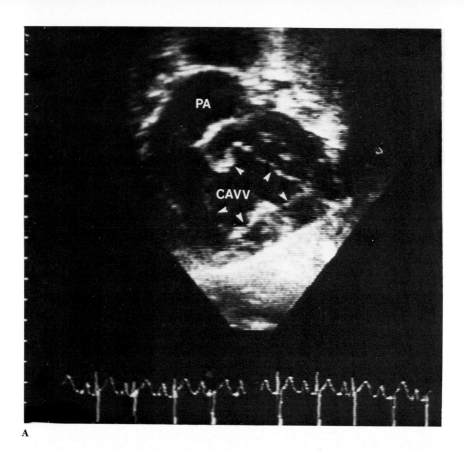

A

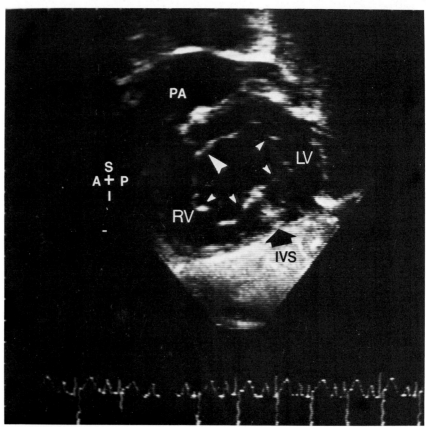

B

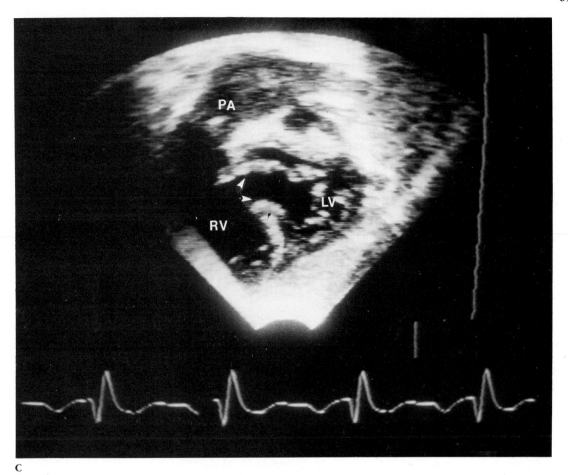

C

Fig. 7-3. (A) Subxiphoid short-axis view of patient with Rastelli type A common atrioventricular valve (*CAVV*) with five leaflets (*arrows*). The superior leaflets do not bridge the ventricular defect. The common atrioventricular valve orifice is equally divided between right (*RV*) and left ventricles (*LV*). (B) Similar view in patient with Rastelli type C atrioventricular septal defect. A large-bridging superior leaflet is seen (*large white arrow*), as well as other leaflets (*small arrows*). (C) Patient with Rastelli type C canal, but smaller ventricular septal defect than patient in B. Bridging portion of superior leaflet forms a straight line as it crosses the interventricular septum. Note the superior and inferior leaflets (*arrows*) are more closely spaced compared with B. *IVS* = interventricular septum; *PA* = pulmonary artery.

CHAPTER 7. Complete Atrioventricular Canal Defects

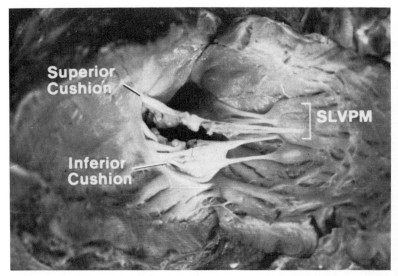

A

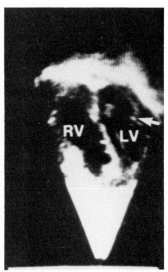

B

Fig. 7-4. (A) Left ventricle (*LV*) opened
from apex and (B) subxiphoid short-
axis of LV in a patient with single papillary muscle. (C and D) The subxiphoid
short-axis view of LV in a patient with a
common atrioventricular valve and normal LV papillary attachments. (E and F)
A single papillary muscle attachment
(*arrows*) in another patient with complete atrioventricular septal defect. *pa*
= pulmonary artery; *RV, rv* = right
ventricle; *SLVPM* = single left ventricular papillary muscle.

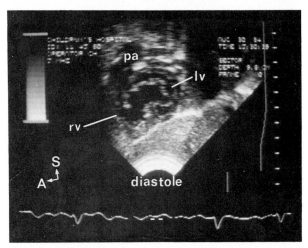

C

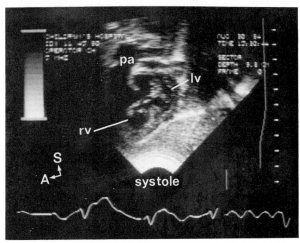

D

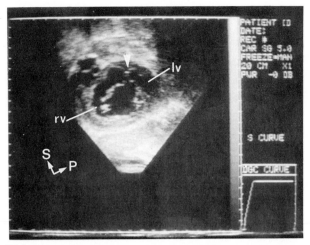

E

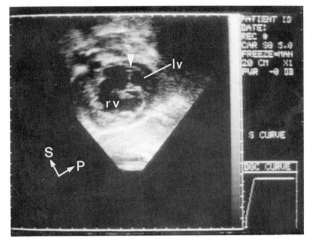

F

EXAMINATION TECHNIQUE

Both atrial septal defects (ASDs) and VSDs can be seen from a single apical or subxiphoid 4-chamber view. The defect may also be seen on subxiphoid or parasternal short-axis views during a sweep from base to apex. Atrioventricular leaflet morphology is best seen from the parasternal and subxiphoid short-axis views because both superior and inferior leaflets are visualized simultaneously (Fig. 7-3). The A-V valves are also seen from the apical and subxiphoid 4-chamber views, but since the leaflets are displayed one at a time (posterior leaflet on inferior angulation, anterior leaflet on superior angulation), care must be taken to identify the leaflets properly by sweeping from one to the other. The position and the number of LV papillary muscles are determined from either precordial or subxiphoid short-axis views.

PROBLEMS

One cannot accurately predict the need for or feasibility of surgical reconstruction of the valve to prevent A-V valve regurgitation. It is difficult to judge leaflet deficiency. Although the cleft or space between the leaflets of the A-V valves can be visualized in diastole, one cannot easily detect poor coaptation between these components in systole. Systolic coaptation of the leaflets relates to leaflet mobility as well as adequacy of leaflet tissue. Also, the presence of additional muscular VSDs may cause significant surgical morbidity if unrecognized.

BIBLIOGRAPHY

Hagler, D. J., Tajik, A. J., and Seward, J. B. Real-time wide-angle sector echocardiography: Atrioventricular canal defects. *Circulation* 59:140, 1979.

Hibi, N., Fukui, Y., Nishimura, K., et al. Cross-sectional echocardiographic study of persistent left superior vena cava. *Am. Heart J.* 100:69, 1980.

Segni, E. P., Bass, J. L., Lucas, R. V., et al. Isolated cleft mitral valve: A variety of congenital mitral regurgitation identified by two-dimensional echocardiography. *Am. J. Cardiol.* 51:927, 1983.

Smallhorn, J. F., Tommasini, G., Anderson, R. H., et al. Assessment of atrioventricular septal defects by two-dimensional echocardiography. *Br. Heart J.* 47:109, 1982.

Smallhorn, J. F., Tommasini, G., and MacCartney, F. J. Two-dimensional echocardiographic assessment of common atrioventricular valves in univentricular hearts. *Br. Heart J.* 46:30, 1981.

Uretzky, G., Puga, F. J., Danielson, G. K., et al. Complete atrioventricular canal associated with tetralogy of Fallot: Morphologic and surgical considerations. *J. Thorac. Cardiovasc. Surg.* 87:756, 1984.

Yoshida, H., Funabashi, T., Nakaya, S., et al. Subxiphoid cross-sectional echocardiographic imaging of the "goose-neck" deformity in endocardial cushion defect. *Circulation* 62:1319, 1980.

CHAPTER 8

Patent Ductus Arteriosus

ANATOMY

A *patent ductus arteriosus* (PDA) is usually short and straight in premature and term newborn infants and long and tortuous in older children. This vessel runs from the junction of the main and left pulmonary arteries (MPA and LPA, respectively) to the inner curvature of the aorta, just distal to the left subclavian artery.

DIAGNOSTIC ECHO
FINDING

The PDA is seen coursing superiorly from the distal MPA superior to the LPA to reach the lesser curvature of the aorta (Figs. 8-1, 8-2). Injection of contrast into the descending aorta will fill the pulmonary artery by retrograde flow, confirming the patency of the vessel. Systemic venous contrast injection may document right-to-left shunting by a PDA in the presence of PA hypertension by passage of contrast from the MPA to the descending aorta. Doppler echocardiography confirms the anatomic findings by showing retrograde or continuous turbulent flow in the MPA.

Fig. 8-1. Suprasternal notch view of patent ductus arteriosus in a patient with transposition of the great arteries. The ductus (*d*) runs between the main pulmonary artery (*MPA*) and the aortic root (*AO*). The left pulmonary artery (*L*) branches from the MPA and courses posteriorly.

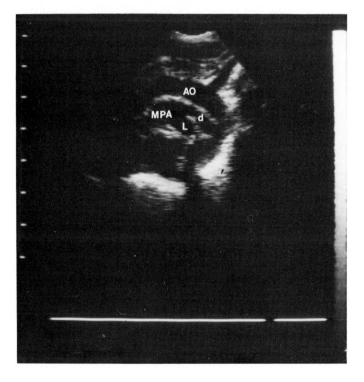

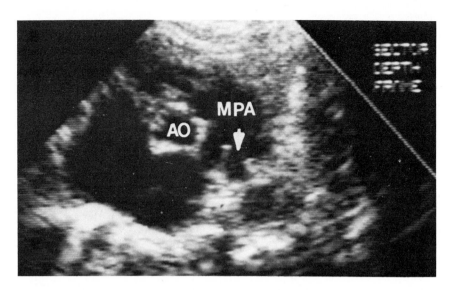

Fig. 8-2. High parasagittal parasternal view of a premature infant with patent ductus arteriosus, which courses to the left of the junction of the main (*MPA*) and left pulmonary arteries (*arrow*). *AO* = aortic root.

EXAMINATION
TECHNIQUE

High suprasternal notch (SSN), high parasagittal parasternal, and subxiphoid short-axis (S4) views demonstrate a PDA (Figs. 8-2, 8-3A, B). The exact position of a PDA depends on the position of the great arteries. It is most easily demonstrated in D-transposition (D-TGA) of the great arteries because the aorta and PA lie parallel to one another. Normally related great arteries are not parallel. Therefore, the PDA must be viewed along the long axis of PA or aortic arch, but not both, simultaneously.

PROBLEMS

Patency of a tortuous or narrowed PDA may be difficult to determine without contrast injection or Doppler examination, whereas a short, wide ductus arteriosus is easy to visualize throughout its course. Premature infants with severe pulmonary disease may have a very limited acoustic window for imaging a PDA. In such patients, demonstration of altered PA flow by Doppler echocardiography has become the most convenient and reliable method for determining the presence of a PDA.

BIBLIOGRAPHY

Gutgesell, H. P., Huhta, J. C., Cohen, M. H., et al. Two-dimensional echocardiographic assessment of pulmonary artery and aortic arch anatomy in cyanotic infants. *J. Am. Coll. Cardiol.* 4:1242, 1984.

Sahn, D. J., and Allen, H. D. Real-time cross-sectional echocardiographic imaging and measurement of the patent ductus arteriosus in infants. *Circulation* 58:343, 1978.

Smallhorn, J. F., Huhta, J. C., Anderson, R. H., et al. Suprasternal cross-sectional echocardiography in assessment of patent ductus arteriosus. *Br. Heart J.* 48:321, 1982.

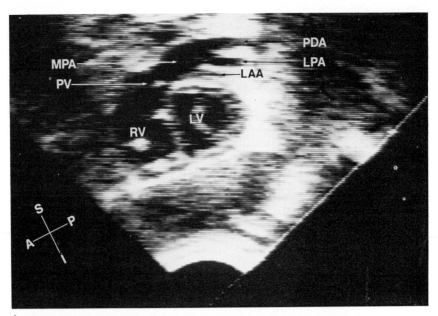

A

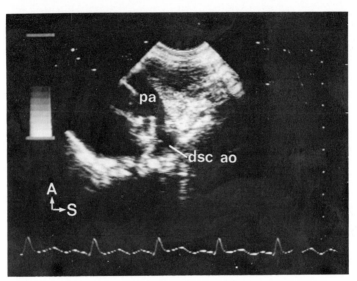

B

Fig. 8-3. (A) Subxiphoid short-axis (of left ventricle [*LV*]) view shows long axis of right ventricle (*RV*) outflow tract and main pulmonary artery (*MPA*, *pa*). The patent ductus arteriosus (*PDA*) continues superiorly and posteriorly from the MPA while the left pulmonary artery (*LPA*) runs directly posteriorly. This view is nearly perpendicular to the aortic arch. (B) High left parasternal view in a nearly sagittal plane demonstrates a PDA coursing between the *pa* and descending aorta (*dsc ao*) in a patient with normally related great arteries. *LAA* = left atrial appendage; *PV* = pulmonary valve.

Total Anomalous Pulmonary Venous Connection

ANATOMY

In *total anomalous pulmonary venous connection* (TAPVC), the pulmonary veins (PVs) do not connect with the left atrium (LA), but drain to the right atrium (RA) directly, indirectly, or via primitive systemic or splanchnic venous pathways (Fig. 9-1A to D). An obligatory right-to-left shunt flows through a patent foramen ovale or atrial septal defect (ASD). The individual PVs often drain into a common horizontal channel lying directly behind the RA and LA. This venous confluence connects the right (RPV) and left (LPV) pulmonary veins. Occasionally the drainage is mixed, with PVs connecting separately to the superior vena cava (SVC), RA, or coronary sinus. Rarely, one or two PVs connect normally to the LA while the remainder drain anomalously. In cases of mixed PV connection, there may be no horizontal channel behind the atria.

In TAPVC to the left-anterior cardinal system, the pathway to the right heart may lead from the horizontal vein to a left vertical vein (persistent left-anterior cardinal vein), and subsequently to the left brachiocephalic vein, which joins the right SVC. Alternatively the PV may connect with the coronary sinus, also a derivative of the left-anterior cardinal system. The PV confluence may connect with right-anterior cardinal system via the azygos vein or an anterior communicating vein. The PVs may also connect to the back wall of the RA.

In the infradiaphragmatic type of drainage, the PVs usually do not form a horizontal confluence; the upper and lower PVs connect separately with a vertical vein crossing the diaphragm in front of the esophagus and running parallel to the inferior vena cava (IVC) on the right and the aorta on the left. The vertical vein may connect with the portal system, ductus venosus, and hepatic veins.

DIAGNOSTIC ECHO FINDINGS

The absence of PV connection to a small LA in the presence of right-to-left bulging of the septum primum at the foramen ovale is often the first indication of the diagnosis (Fig. 9-2A, B).

The prerequisite finding for TAPVC is the identification of PV connection to the systemic veins, coronary sinus, or RA, rather than to the LA. All four PVs and their connections must be identified in order to accurately diagnose the mixed type of anomalous PV connection.

INDIRECT FINDINGS

Documentation of the right-to-left shunt at the atrial level is a nonspecific supportive finding. PV drainage via the SVC, IVC, or coronary sinus usually causes dilation of these structures. RA and right ventricular (RV) dilation are usually, but not invariably, present.

Fig. 9-1. Diagrams depict total anomalous pulmonary venous connection to the superior vena cava (*SVC*) (A), the left-anterior cardinal system (B), the coronary sinus (C), and the portal system (D). Some patients have a mixed type of drainage that combines two or more of these types of connections. *IVC* = inferior vena cava; *LA* = left atrium; *RA* = right atrium.

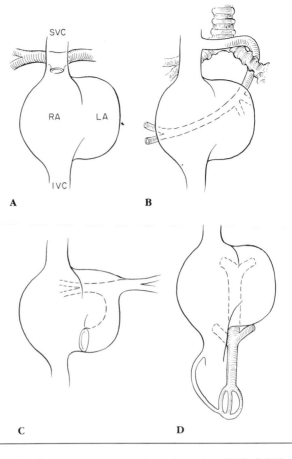

A

B

C

D

Fig. 9-2. Subxiphoid 4-chamber views of normal patient (A) and patient with total anomalous pulmonary venous connection (B). (A) The upper right pulmonary vein (*RPV*) entrance of the left atrium (*LA*). The position of the flap valve of the foramen ovale (*arrow*) moves both right and left during the cardiac cycle, here shown bulging toward the right atrium (*RA*). (B) The horizontal confluence of pulmonary veins (*VC*) lies behind the atrial cavity, but does not connect with the LA. The flap valve of the foramen ovale (*short arrow*) bulges into the LA throughout the cardiac cycle because of the obligatory right-to-left shunt at that level.

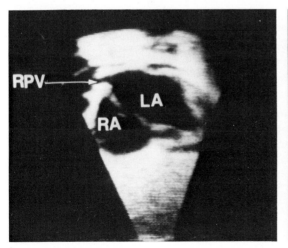

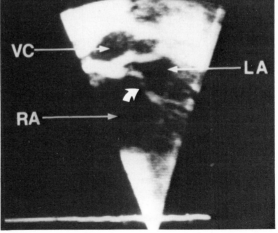

A

B

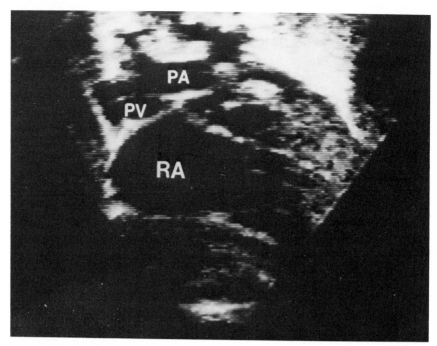

A

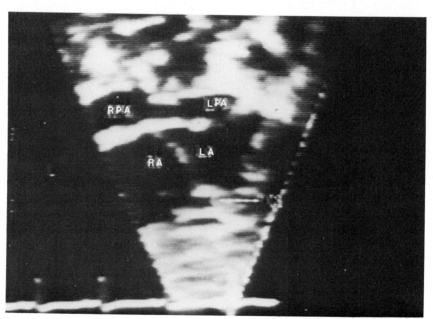

B

Fig. 9-3. (A) Superior angulation from subxiphoid 4-chamber view shows right pulmonary vein (*PV*) running right to left beneath the right pulmonary artery (*PA*). (B) Subxiphoid 4-chamber view showing horizontal venous channel connecting the right and left PVs as they lie behind the atrial cavity. The vein does not connect with the left atrium (*LA*). *LPA* = left pulmonary artery; *RA* = right atrium; *RPA* = right pulmonary artery.

PART II. Shunt Lesions

EXAMINATION
TECHNIQUE

There is no standard method for tracing the PV pathways because of their unlimited anatomic variation. It is simplest to identify the bifurcation of the right and left pulmonary arteries (RPA and LPA, respectively) from sub-xiphoid long-axis views and sweep the transducer inferiorly until the PVs are visualized (Fig. 9-3A, B). If a vertical vein connects this horizontal PV with the left brachiocephalic or right SVC, this structure may be viewed in long axis from suprasternal views (Fig. 9-4). Supradiaphragmatic TAPVC to the right SVC may be demonstrated from parasagittal subxiphoid and high right parasternal views that display the long axis of the SVC (S1) as seen in Figure 9-5A, B.

PVs entering the coronary sinus are displayed from subxiphoid and apical 4-chamber views or subxiphoid short-axis views (Fig. 9-6A to C). These views may also demonstrate PV return directly to the RA (Fig. 9-6D).

Fig. 9-4. Suprasternal notch coronal plane of patient with supracardiac type of total anomalous pulmonary venous connection (*TAPVC*) demonstrating horizontal venous confluence (*VC*), vertical vein (*VV*), and innominate vein. The connection between the VV and innominate vein is obliterated by bright echoes representing air in the left mainstem bronchus. Compare this with Figure 9-1B. *AO* = aorta; *HV* = horizontal vein; *PA* = pulmonary artery.

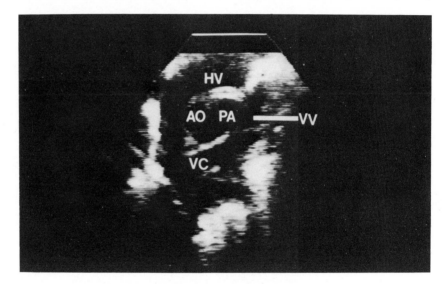

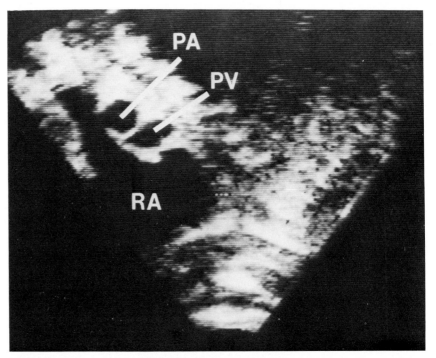

A

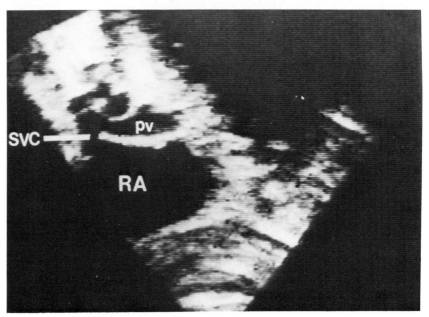

B

Fig. 9-5. (A) Subxiphoid parasagittal view (S1) demonstrates long axis of superior vena cava (*SVC*) as it courses inferiorly to enter right atrium (*RA*). The right pulmonary artery (*PA*) and pulmonary vein (*PV, pv*) are seen in cross section as they pass behind the SVC. (B) Slight angulation from previous view shows direct entrance of pv into SVC. Compare this with Figure 9-1A.

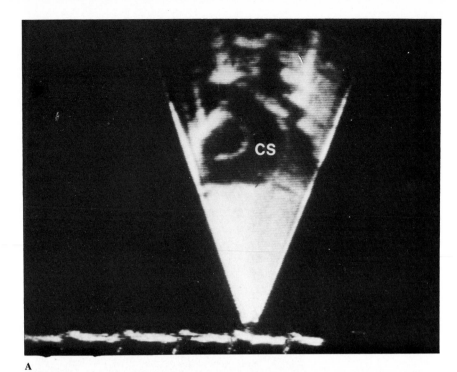

A

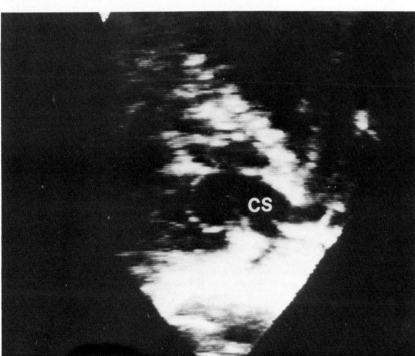

B

Fig. 9-6. (A) Low subxiphoid 4-chamber view illustrating total anomalous pulmonary venous connection to the coronary sinus (*CS*). A dilated CS carries pulmonary venous return from the posterior atrial wall into the floor of the right atrium. Compare this illustration with Figure 9-1C. (B) Subxiphoid short-axis view with inferior angulation. The lower pulmonary vein entrance to the CS is shown.

CHAPTER 9. Total Anomalous Pulmonary Venous Connection

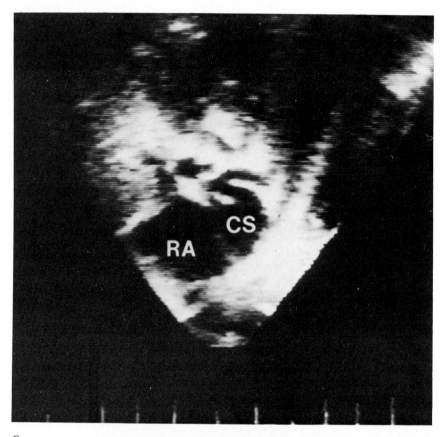

C

(**Fig. 9-6** continued)
(C) Subxiphoid short-axis view with
superior angulation showing the entrance of upper pulmonary veins to CS.
(D) Right subxiphoid 4-chamber view
demonstrating direct pulmonary venous connection (*pvc*) to the back wall
of the right atrium. *la* = left atrium; *RA*,
ra = right atrium.

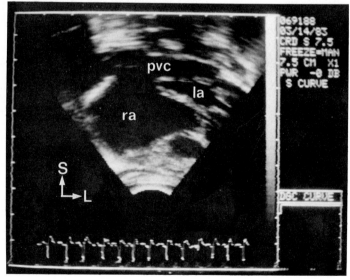

D

The vertical vein in the infradiaphragmatic type of TAPVC is optimally visualized from the subxiphoid approach. With the sector plane in the sagittal plane of the body, the transducer is inclined rightward to display the IVC, then leftward to display the length of the descending aorta. The anomalous vertical vein is a prominent structure, displayed along its long axis as it lies behind the heart and in front of the esophagus, situated between the IVC (to the right) and the aorta (to the left) (Fig. 9-7A). Rotating the transducer 90° to a transverse section of the trunk at the level of the diaphragm will display the vertical vein in cross section. Superior angulation of the transducer from this position will allow the vertical channel to be traced back to its PV tributaries (Fig. 9-7B).

Injection of contrast into a systemic vein documents a right-to-left shunt at the atrial level and fills all vessels except the PV system. This technique may be used to verify the identity of PVs. Doppler echocardiography sampling within the structure will also identify a venous flow pattern toward the heart.

Fig. 9-7. (A) Subxiphoid parasagittal plane in a patient with infradiaphragmatic total anomalous pulmonary venous connection. Vertical vein (*VV*) lies between inferior vena cava and descending aorta (*AO*) as it descends behind the heart and past the diaphragm. Compare this with Figure 9-1D. (B) Subxiphoid plane horizontal to trunk, imaging posterior to the atrial cavity, showing gull-wing pattern of right and left pulmonary veins joining the VV. Upper and lower veins are visualized separately. *LA* = left atrium; *RA* = right atrium.

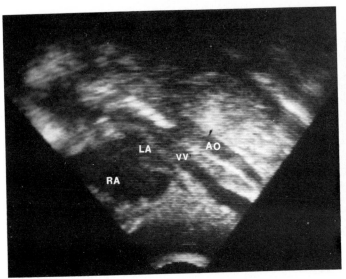

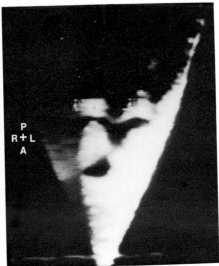

A

B

CHAPTER 9. Total Anomalous Pulmonary Venous Connection

PROBLEMS

The important differential diagnosis for TAPVC is persistent fetal circulation (primary PA hypertension of the newborn). The clinical picture might be quite similar in these lesions; both have a right-to-left shunt at the atrial level and RV dilatation. The pulmonary systolic time intervals usually indicate PA hypertension in both lesions. Because of these similarities, it is necessary to identify the PV connections positively in order to make the proper diagnosis.

Excellent axial and lateral resolution is required to successfully trace venous connections within the posterior and superior mediastinum. Unfortunately, many commonly used transducers are tightly focused at depths required for examination of the heart, but the beam width increases considerably at the depth of the PVs and their connections. Poor resolution may cause structures in near proximity to appear to connect: This is a major source of error since the horizontal PV confluence usually lies close to the back wall of the atrium.

It is possible to mistake the bifurcating PA for a horizontal PV. The PAs should be identified as separate structures by sweeping the transducer superiorly from the long axis position that demonstrates the PVs.

In the supracardiac type of PV drainage to the left-anterior cardinal system, the vertical vein may not be visualized in its entirety because (1) its course may be tortuous, connecting the PVs in the posterior mediastinum with an extremely anterior innominate vein, (2) the course of the vertical vein may vary, passing anterior or posterior to the LPA, or (3) the vein passes over the left main stem bronchus or its tributaries. Intense echo reflections from air in these structures shadow the vein, creating the deceptive appearance of discontinuity.

In some patients with TAPVC, extreme curvature of the interatrial septum into the LA may create the impression of a vessel entering the left superior aspect of the LA (see Fig. 9-2B).

BIBLIOGRAPHY

Aziz, K. U., Paul, M. H., Bharati, S., et al. Echocardiographic features of total anomalous pulmonary venous drainage to the coronary sinus. *Am. J. Cardiol.* 42: 108, 1978.

Delisle, G., Ando, M., Calder, A. L., et al. Total anomalous pulmonary venous connection. Report of 93 autopsied cases with emphasis on diagnostic and surgical consideration. *Am. Heart J.* 91:99, 1976.

Orsmond, G. S., Ruttenburg, H. D., Bessinger, F. B., et al. Echocardiographic features of total anomalous pulmonary venous connection to the coronary sinus. *Am. J. Cardiol.* 41:108, 1978.

Pickoff, A. S., Sequeira, R., Ferrer, P. L., et al. Pulsed Doppler echocardiographic findings in total anomalous pulmonary venous drainage to the coronary sinus. *Cathet. Cardiovasc. Diagn.* 6:247, 1980.

Sahn, D. J., Allen, H. D., Lange, L. W., et al. Cross-sectional echocardiographic diagnosis of the sites of total anomalous pulmonary venous drainage. *Circulation* 60:1317, 1979.

PART II. Shunt Lesions

Skovrane, K. J., Tuma, S., Urbancova, D., et al. Range-gated pulsed Doppler echocardiographic diagnosis of supracardiac total anomalous pulmonary venous drainage. *Circulation* 61:841, 1980.

Smallhorn, J. F., Sutherland, G. F., Tommasini, G., et al. Assessment of total anomalous pulmonary venous connection with two-dimensional echocardiography. *Br. Heart J.* 46:613, 1981.

Snider, A. R., Silverman, N. H., Turley, K., and Ebert, P. Evaluation of infradiaphragmatic total anomalous pulmonary venous connection with two-dimensional echocardiography. *Circulation* 66:1129, 1982.

Stevenson, J. G., Kawabori, I., and Guntheroth, W. G. Pulsed Doppler echocardiographic detection of total anomalous pulmonary venous return: Resolution of left atrial line. *Am. J. Cardiol.* 44:115, 1979.

Vick, G. W., III, Huhta, J. C., and Gutgesell, H. P. Assessment of the ductus arteriosus in preterm infants, utilizing suprasternal two-dimensional/Doppler echocardiography. *J. Am. Coll. Cardiol.* 5:973, 1985.

Partial Anomalous Pulmonary Venous Connection

ANATOMY

In *partial anomalous pulmonary venous connection* (PAPVC), one or more of the pulmonary veins (PVs), (most commonly the upper right pulmonary veins [RPVs]) enter the right lateral border of the right atrium (RA) at the superior vena cava (SVC) junction or, in some cases, higher on the SVC. In a group of lesions known as scimitar syndrome, upper or lower RPVs may drain to the inferior vena cava (IVC), in association with anomalies of the pulmonary arteries (PAs). Ipsilateral drainage of the right- and left-sided PVs occurs in patients with heterotaxia and common atrium.

The clinical presentation of PAPVC is similar to that of atrial septal defect (ASD). Partial anomalous pulmonary venous connection (PAPVC) may be an isolated lesion but is commonly associated with the sinus venosus type of ASD.

DIAGNOSTIC ECHO FINDINGS

Visualization of the entrance of a PV into the RA or SVC is the most definitive finding for this anomaly (Fig. 10-1).

INDIRECT FINDINGS

In a patient with typical clinical features for right ventricular (RV) volume overload, the inability to demonstrate an ASD should raise the question of isolated PAPVC. The strength of this suspicion lies heavily on the completeness with which the atrial septum is displayed.

EXAMINATION TECHNIQUE

Entrance of the PVs into the RA or SVC can be displayed from subxiphoid or apical 4-chamber views. A subxiphoid long-axis position with superior angulation (L3) has the advantage of demonstrating the SVC as well as the right lateral border of the RA. Suprasternal notch (SSN) and right sternal border parasagittal views, which display the long axis of the SVC, are very useful for displaying PVs connecting to the high cava or midcava. It is sometimes difficult to define the exact relationship of the PVs to the atria when the adjacent portion of the atrial septum is absent (i.e., sinus venosus defect). The atrial septum should be examined carefully by multiple transducer sweeps to detect associated ASDs (see Chap. 5).

PITFALLS

The major diagnostic problems are purely technical rather than conceptual, relating to the quality of imaging of the posterior mediastinum, RA border, and SVC. These areas are usually well seen in the small child, but visualiza-

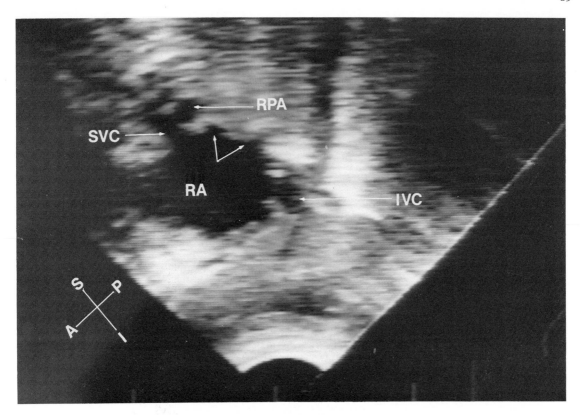

Fig. 10-1. Subxiphoid short-axis, parasagittal, or caval view of a patient with return of the right pulmonary veins to the back wall of the right atrium (*RA*). Entrances of pulmonary veins are marked (*arrows*), the upper vein to the high atrial wall near the junction with the superior vena cava (*SVC*), the lower to the midposterior atrium. The right pulmonary artery (*RPA*) is seen in cross section as it passes behind the SVC above the pulmonary veins. *IVC* = inferior vena cava.

tion becomes increasingly difficult with advancing age and size because of a limited acoustic window.

When a sinus venosus–type ASD is seen, the examiner should take special care to define the entrance of the PVs.

BIBLIOGRAPHY   Damlowicz, D., and Kronzon, I. Use of contrast echocardiography in the diagnosis of partial anomalous pulmonary venous connection. *Am. J. Cardiol.* 42:248, 1979.

CHAPTER 10. Partial Anomalous Pulmonary Venous Connection

CHAPTER 11

Aorticopulmonary Window

ANATOMY

In *aorticopulmonary window*, there is incomplete septation of the aorticopulmonary sac into the ascending aorta and main pulmonary artery (MPA) components. The defect lies above the semilunar valves and below the bifurcation of the pulmonary artery (PA) and is often large. Patent ductus arteriosus (PDA) occasionally accompanies this lesion.

DIAGNOSTIC ECHO FINDINGS

The defect must be directly visualized from at least two views that simultaneously display the long or short axis of both great arteries. The PA, left atrium (LA), and left ventricle (LV) are dilated. Since the clinical presentation of aorticopulmonary defect is similar to a large ventricular septal defect (VSD), the appearance of an intact ventricular septum is supportive of the diagnosis of the arterial defect. Visualization of a PDA does not make the presence of an aorticopulmonary defect less likely. This lesion can be differentiated from hemitruncus because, in aorticopulmonary window, the right and left pulmonary arteries (RPA and LPA, respectively) are continuous with each other and with the MPA.

EXAMINATION TECHNIQUE

The defect may be viewed from a high parasternal short-axis view of the PA and ascending aorta (Fig. 11-1) or from a subxiphoid long-axis view of the LV and ascending aorta (Fig. 11-2). Since the wall between the aorta and PA spirals and lies roughly parallel to the echo beam from both views, careful sweeping must be performed to rule out artifactual dropout.

PROBLEMS

Because aorticopulmonary window is rare and easily confused clinically with VSD, the great arteries may not be adequately scanned to visualize the entire aorticopulmonary septum. Moreover, the truncal septum is curved and positioned so that it is difficult to view perpendicularly. Nevertheless, the defect is usually large and can be clearly displayed if the examination is performed with the diagnosis in mind. False dropout of the medial wall of the main pulmonary artery may be present in one view, such as the transverse parasternal view; therefore, it is important to verify the presence of a defect in more than one plane.

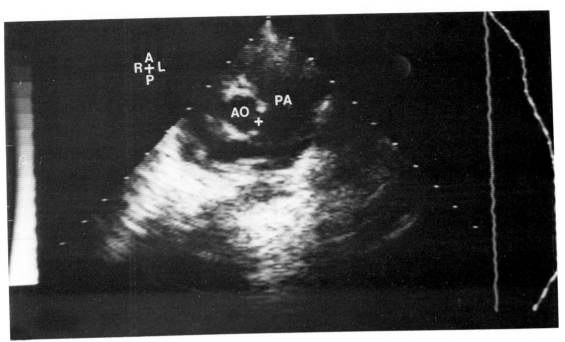

Fig. 11-1. High parasternal short-axis view of great arteries shows defect between aorta (*AO*) and pulmonary artery (*PA*) (+). Because artifactual echo dropout is common in this area, the presence of a defect must be confirmed in another plane.

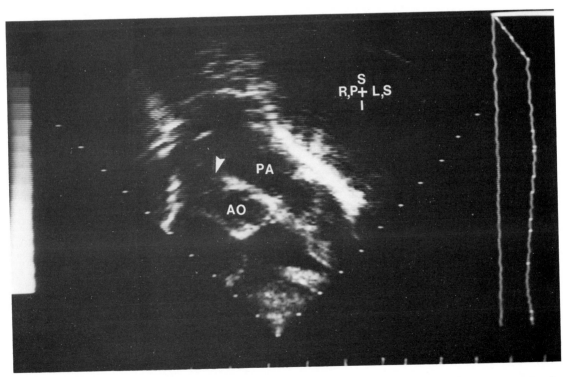

Fig. 11-2. Subxiphoid long-axis view with counterclockwise rotation demonstrates ascending portions of aorta (*AO*) and pulmonary artery (*PA*) with defect (*arrow*). The upper margin of the defect is not clearly seen on this single frame but was apparent in real time.

BIBLIOGRAPHY

Neufeld, H. N., Lester, R. G., Adams, P. J., et al. Aorticopulmonary septal defect. *Am. J. Cardiol.* 9:12, 1962.

Rice, M. J., Seward, J. B., Hagler, D. J., et al. Visualization of aorticopulmonary window by two-dimensional echocardiography. *Mayo Clin. Proc.* 57:482, 1982.

Richardson, J. V., Doty, D. B., Rossi, N. P., et al. The spectrum of anomalies of aorticopulmonary septation. *J. Thorac. Cardiovasc. Surg.* 78:21, 1979.

Smallhorn, J. F., Anderson, B. H., and MacCartney, F. J. Two-dimensional echocardiographic assessment of communications between ascending aorta and pulmonary trunk or individual pulmonary arteries. *Br. Heart J.* 47:563, 1982.

CHAPTER 12

Anomalous Left Coronary Artery

ANATOMY

Anomalous origin of the left coronary artery from the main pulmonary artery (MPA) is a rare abnormality that often presents with low output state or severe congestive heart failure in infancy. The left coronary artery may arise from any aspect of the MPA. It runs in the atrioventricular (A-V) groove, passing close to the left side of the aortic root. In older patients, the left coronary artery is large because of a left-to-right shunt from the right coronary artery, through collaterals to the left coronary artery and then to the pulmonary artery (PA). Ischemia or infarction of the anterolateral left ventricular (LV) wall is often present.

DIAGNOSTIC ECHO FINDINGS

The normal origin of the left coronary artery may be demonstrated from parasternal short- and long-axis (with leftward angulation) views and subxiphoid long-axis views (Figs. 12-1, 12-2). The origin of the anomalous left coronary artery may be visualized from long- or short-axis views of the PA (Fig. 12-3). Simple absence of the left coronary artery from its usual origin at the left sinus of the aortic root does not distinguish this lesion from single coronary artery. Segmental wall motion abnormality involving the anterolateral free wall of the LV indicates ischemia or infarction.

Doppler examination reveals continuous turbulent flow in the MPA near the coronary orifice. In addition, Doppler examination may reveal a mitral regurgitant jet in the left atrium (LA) as a consequence of papillary muscle dysfunction.

EXAMINATION TECHNIQUES

Difficulty in displaying the origin of the left coronary artery in its usual location in the setting of low cardiac output and LV dysfunction in the infant should prompt an intensive search for the origin of the coronary artery from the MPA. Since the vessel may arise from any aspect of the PA, all sides of the PA should be inspected from parasternal and subxiphoid views. Doppler examination should be performed with the sample volume in the abnormal vessel and its pulmonary orifice as well as in the LA to seek evidence of mitral regurgitation. In older children, dilatation of the coronary arteries may be the first clue to the diagnosis.

PROBLEMS

The anomalous left coronary artery may lie very close to the left aortic sinus of the aortic root. If lateral resolution is poor, the lumina of these two structures may merge so that the coronary artery appears to rise from the aortic root. Excellent resolution is required to adequately display abnormalities of vessels as small as the coronary arteries.

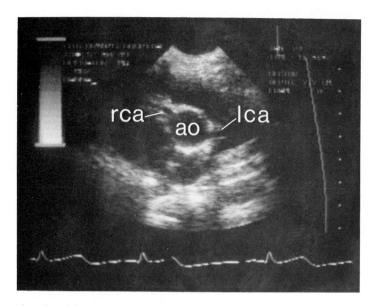

Fig. 12-1. This is a parasternal short-axis view of a patient with normal origin of the left coronary artery (*lca*) from the left aortic sinus. The right coronary artery (*rca*) can be seen rising from the anterior aspect of the aortic root (*ao*).

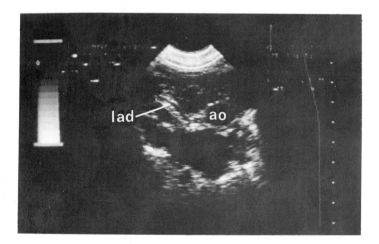

Fig. 12-2. Parasternal long-axis view of normal left coronary artery and branch left anterior descending coronary artery (*lad*) arising from the aortic root (*ao*).

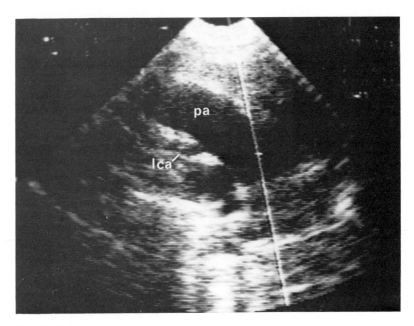

Fig. 12-3. Parasternal long-axis view
with left angulation shows connection
between the left coronary (*lca*) and
main pulmonary arteries (*pa*).

BIBLIOGRAPHY

Caldwell, R. F., Hurwitz, R. A., Girod, D. A., et al. Two-dimensional echocardiographic differentiation of anomalous left coronary artery from congestive cardiomyopathy. *Am. J. Cardiol.* 106:710, 1983.

Fisher, E. A., Sepehri, B., Lendrum, B., Luken, J., and Levitsky, S. Two-dimensional echocardiographic visualization of the left coronary artery in anomalous origins of the left coronary artery from the pulmonary artery. *Circulation* 63:3:698, 1981.

Robinson, P. J., Sullivan, I. D., Kumping, V., et al. Anomalous origin of the left coronary artery from the pulmonary trunk: Potential for false negative diagnosis with cross-sectional echocardiography. *Br. Heart J.* 52:272, 1984.

Terai, M., Nagai, Y., and Toba, T. Cross-sectional echocardiographic findings of anomalous left coronary artery from pulmonary artery. *Br. Heart J.* 50:104, 1983.

Obstructive Lesions

Ebstein's Anomaly of the Tricuspid Valve

ANATOMY

Ebstein's anomaly of the tricuspid valve has a wide range of anatomic variation. In its more common form, the proximal attachment of the septal tricuspid leaflet is displaced inferiorly and leftward toward the right ventricular (RV) apex (Fig. 13-1). This displacement may be so mild that it involves only a portion of the septal leaflet or so severe that the entire tricuspid valve is displaced leftward and superiorly, lying between the inflow and outflow portions of the RV. When displacement involves only the septal leaflet, the anterior leaflet is usually large and saillike, reaching from the true annulus to coapt with the distal edge of the displaced septal leaflet. The displacement of the tricuspid valve into the RV leaves a large right atrial (RA) chamber with ventricular myocardium forming the lateral walls inferiorly (atrialized RV). The RV inflow is reciprocally smaller.

Tricuspid leaflets and chordal attachments may be nearly normal, but are more commonly thickened and fused. The anterior leaflet may be either large and saillike or foreshortened. Occasionally a portion of the tricuspid valve apparatus may cause subpulmonary obstruction. The tricuspid valve may be stenosed or regurgitant or may function in a nearly normal fashion. RA enlargement is variable, depending on tricuspid valve function and decompression via a patent foramen ovale or atrial septal defect (ASD). Severe dilatation of the RA and the atrialized portion of the RV compresses the left ventricle (LV).

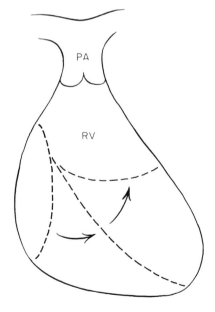

Fig. 13-1. Diagram of right ventricle (*RV*) in Ebstein's anomaly of the tricuspid valve. The true tricuspid annulus is in the normal position, but the line of attachment of the septal tricuspid leaflet is displaced toward the apex. Arrows point to differing degrees of displacement of the septal leaflet attachment as designated by dotted lines. *PA* = pulmonary artery.

DIAGNOSTIC ECHO
FINDINGS

The sine qua non of Ebstein's anomaly is displacement of the septal tricuspid leaflet (Figs. 13-2, 13-3). This leaflet is usually severely foreshortened so that leaflet motion cannot be easily discerned. Prominent motion of a large saillike anterior leaflet is often the first and most easily recognized feature (Fig. 13-4). This finding will not be present in patients with the displacement of the entire tricuspid valve. In its most severe form, the valve may be represented by a membrane between the inflow and outflow portions of the RV as shown in Figure 13-5A, B. As a result of severe displacement of the leaflet(s), the tricuspid orifice faces the pulmonary outflow.

Fig. 13-2. Apical 4-chamber view of Ebstein's anomaly shows marked displacement of septal tricuspid attachment to the interventricular septum (*large arrow*), relative to the attachment of the mitral leaflet (*small arrow*). The right atrium (*RA*) is very large and includes the atrialized portion of the right ventricle (*RV*). *LA* = left atrium; *LV* = left ventricle.

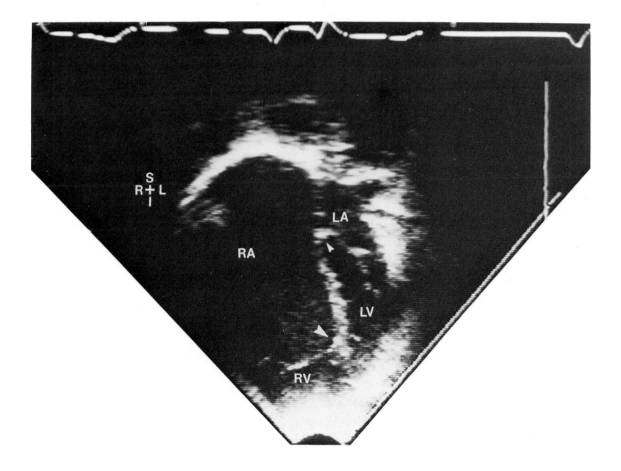

CHAPTER 13. Ebstein's Anomaly of the Tricuspid Valve

Usually, the RA is remarkably dilated, its lower walls formed by the atrialized RV. Conversely, the RV is smaller than normal.

A right-to-left shunt at the atrial level is usually, but not invariably, present and may be demonstrated by systemic venous contrast injection.

Tricuspid regurgitation, if present, may be demonstrated by Doppler examination or contrast injection.

Delayed tricuspid closure (>0.06 sec after mitral closure) is a specific but insensitive indicator of Ebstein's anomaly.

EXAMINATION
TECHNIQUE

From an apical 4-chamber view, the attachment of the septal tricuspid leaflet must be located relative to a fixed intracardiac landmark such as the crux of the heart. Displacement of septal leaflet may also be assessed by noting its position relative to the aortic annulus in subxiphoid long- or short-axis position. Superior displacement toward the RV outflow tract in severe cases is best shown on subxiphoid long-axis views of the RV outflow tract.

PROBLEMS

Diagnostic difficulties are usually encountered only with extremes of severity. Diagnosis of the most subtle form of anomaly is difficult because there are no values for the smallest amount of leaflet displacement consistent with Ebstein's anomaly. In some patients, only the inferior portion of the septal tricuspid leaflet is displaced apically, so that display of only the more superior portion of that leaflet may lead to a false-negative diagnosis.

In the most severe form of this disease, the entire valve is displaced. Therefore, the anterior tricuspid leaflet is diminished rather than elongated. Simple awareness of this form of the anomaly is sufficient to prevent a false-negative diagnosis.

BIBLIOGRAPHY

Gussenhoren, W. J., Spitaels, S. E. C., Bom, N., et al. Echocardiographic criteria for Ebstein's anomaly of the tricuspid valve. *Br. Heart J.* 43:31, 1980.

Hirschklan, M. J., Sahn, D. J., Hagan, A. D., et al. Cross-sectional echocardiographic features of Ebstein's anomaly of the tricuspid valve. *Am. J. Cardiol.* 40:400, 1977.

Matsumoto, M., Matsuo, H., Nagata, S., et al. Visualization of Ebstein's anomaly of the tricuspid valve by two-dimensional and standard echocardiography. *Circulation* 53:69, 1976.

Ports, T. A., Silverman, N. H., and Schiller, N. B. Two-dimensional echocardiographic assessment of Ebstein's anomaly. *Circulation* 58:336, 1978.

Shiina, A., Seward, J. B., Edwards, W. D., et al. Two-dimensional echocardiographic spectrum of Ebstein's anomaly. Detailed anatomic assessment. *J. Am. Coll. Cardiol.* 3:356, 1984.

Shiina, A., Seward, J. B., Tajik, A. J., et al. Two-dimensional echocardiographic surgical correlation in Ebstein's anomaly: Preoperative determination of patients requiring tricuspid valve plication vs. replacement. *Circulation* 68:534, 1983.

CHAPTER 14

Tricuspid Atresia

ANATOMY

In tricuspid atresia, there is usually no vestige of a right atrial (RA)–right ventricular (RV) connection (Fig. 14-1). Rarely there is a recognizable tricuspid annulus and an imperforate membrane. The only means of egress from the RA is an interatrial communication. A single atrioventricular (A-V) valve, the mitral valve, is situated to the left of the atrial septum. The RV inflow tract is absent or underdeveloped. The size of the RV outflow tract may be small to normal, depending on the size of the interventricular communication. The left ventricle (LV) is usually dilated and may function abnormally, particularly in older patients. The conotruncal anatomy may be similar to tetralogy of Fallot with infundibular (subpulmonary) stenosis (see Chap. 27). The great vessels are most often normally related, but may be transposed. When tricuspid atresia is associated with D-transposition of the great arteries (D-TGA), the possibility of juxtaposition of the atrial appendages or obstructive lesions of the aortic arch should be investigated.

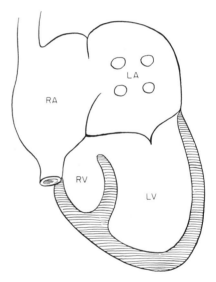

Fig. 14-1. Diagram of tricuspid atresia depicts absent right atrial–right ventricular connection. Exit from the right atrium (*RA*) is via a patent foramen ovale. The mitral valve is to the left of the interatrial septum. The left ventricle (*LV*) is dilated and the right ventricle (*RV*) hypoplastic. Only a portion of the right atrioventricular sulcus is seen here. *LA* = left atrium.

DIAGNOSTIC ECHO
FINDINGS

In tricuspid atresia, there is no A-V valve to the right of the interatrial septum in a patient with normal ventricular looping (Fig. 14-2). The single A-V valve to the left of the interatrial septum is a morphologic mitral valve (i.e., there is a deep septal leaflet separated from the interventricular septum [IVS] by an outflow tract; the valve attaches to two free-wall papillary muscles).

There is no RA-to-RV connection. The only route for egress of blood from the RA is via a patent foramen ovale or an atrial septal defect (ASD) (Fig. 14-3). This right-to-left shunting is indicated by bulging of the septum primum into the left atrium (LA) throughout the cardiac cycle, but may be documented by contrast injection into a systemic vein, showing passage of bubbles from the RA to the LA. In tricuspid atresia, the contrast first appears in the anterior RV outflow chamber during systole since it fills only from the LV during ejection.

Fig. 14-2. Apical 4-chamber view of a patient with tricuspid atresia. A single atrioventricular valve, the mitral valve, is present. *LA* = left atrium; *LV* = left ventricle; *RA* = right atrium.

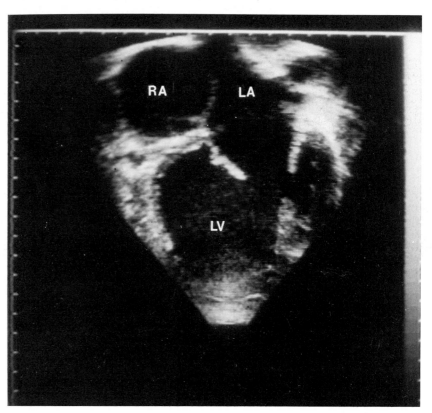

The RV inflow appears atretic or is not seen at all from apical 4-chamber or subxiphoid views.

EXAMINATION TECHNIQUE

The apical and subxiphoid 4-chamber views display the crux of the heart and are, therefore, the best views for demonstrating tricuspid atresia. The RV outflow tract and VSD are usually best displayed from subxiphoid or parasternal short-axis views.

Doppler examination or systemic venous contrast injection while imaging both atria demonstrates the right-to-left shunting at the atrial level.

Fig. 14-3. Subxiphoid 4-chamber view of a patient with tricuspid atresia showing patent foramen ovale (*arrow*) with the flap valve deviated into the left atrium (*LA*). *LV* = left ventricle; *RA* = right atrium.

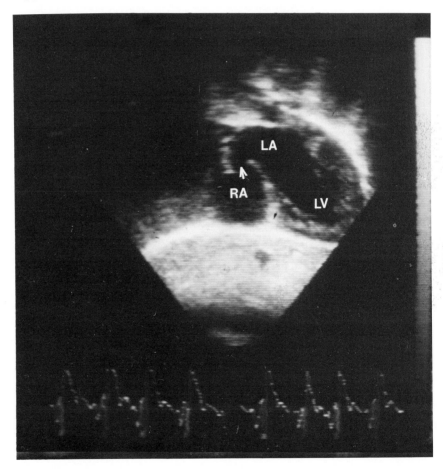

PROBLEMS

The appearance of tricuspid atresia is usually obvious and does not offer major diagnostic difficulties. This diagnosis may be distinguished from other lesions with a common A-V valve because the interatrial septum is entirely to one side of the sole A-V valve (whereas the interatrial septum straddles the orifice of a common A-V valve) and from mitral atresia by the morphology of the A-V valve and ventricle.

In severe forms of hypoplastic right heart with pulmonary atresia and hypoplastic tricuspid annulus, it may be difficult to determine the patency of the tricuspid valve. Here, contrast injection may indicate whether or not the RV fills from the tricuspid valve during diastole.

BIBLIOGRAPHY

Beppu, S., Nimura, Y., Tamai, M., et al. Two-dimensional echocardiography in diagnosing tricuspid atresia. *Br. Heart J.* 40:1174, 1978.

Bharati, S., McAllister, H. A., Tatooles, C. J., et al. Anatomic variations in underdeveloped right ventricle related to tricuspid atresia and stenosis. *J. Thorac. Cardiovasc. Surg.* 72:383, 1976.

Bierman, F. Z., Fellows, K., and Williams, R. G. Prospective identification of ventricular septal defects in infancy using subxiphoid two-dimensional echocardiography. *Circulation* 62:807, 1980.

Hagler, D. J., Tajik, A. J., Seward, J. B., et al. Real-time wide-angle sector echocardiography: Atrioventricular canal defects. *Circulation* 59:140, 1979.

Seward, J. B., Tajik, A. J., Hagler, D. J., et al. Echocardiographic spectrum of tricuspid atresia. *Mayo Clin. Proc.* 91:100, 1978.

Takahashi, O., Eshaghpour, E., and Kotler, M. N. Tricuspid and pulmonic valve echoes in tricuspid and pulmonary atresia. *Chest* 76:437, 1979.

Hypoplastic Right Heart: Critical Pulmonic Stenosis and Pulmonary Atresia with Intact Ventricular Septum

ANATOMY

The hypoplastic right heart syndrome with critical or complete pulmonary outflow obstruction is characterized by tricuspid and pulmonary valve abnormalities. The size of the right ventricle (RV) ranges from nearly normal in some infants with critical pulmonary stenosis to a small, slitlike space in patients with pulmonary atresia, intact ventricular septum, and severe tricuspid stenosis.

The size of the tricuspid annulus generally reflects the degree of RV hypoplasia. The tricuspid valve may be thickened, poorly differentiated from the RV endocardium, fused, and foreshortened and may have abnormally short and thickened chordae tendineae.

The RV outflow tract is usually diminutive. The pulmonary valve is represented by a membrane that may move up and down during the cardiac cycle. In patients with critical pulmonary stenosis, an exceedingly small, pinhole orifice is present. The main and branch pulmonary arteries (PAs) are usually hypoplastic, and the patent ductus arteriosus (PDA), if present, is narrow and tortuous.

Right-to-left flow through a patent foramen ovale or atrial septal defect (ASD) is invariably present in these patients.

DIAGNOSTIC ECHO FINDINGS

Hypoplasia of RV inflow and outflow tracts, associated with a domed or immobile valve or membrane across the pulmonary annulus, is characteristic of this group of anomalies (Figs. 15-1, 15-2, 15-3). It is very difficult to distinguish the atretic from the minimally patent valve by visualization alone.

Attempts to recognize antegrade flow through the valve by Doppler examination or contrast injection are usually successful, but are limited by the small size of the PAs. Usually, however, a high-velocity jet during systole may be detected by Doppler examination in the main pulmonary artery (MPA) in patients with critical pulmonary stenosis, while in pulmonary atresia, the flow pattern in the PA and branches is retrograde and continuous.

The tricuspid valve is often thickened and immobile, but rarely domes in diastole. The sizes of the tricuspid annulus and leaflet are roughly proportional to the size of the RV.

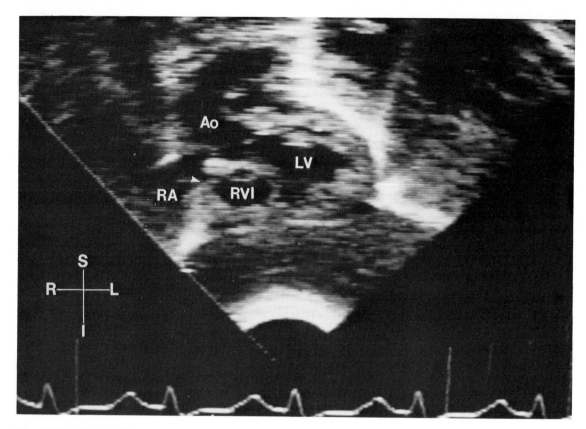

Fig. 15-1. Subxiphoid long-axis view (L3) in a patient with critical pulmonary stenosis and hypoplastic right heart. Dense, white echoes (*arrow*) between right atrium (*RA*) and right ventricular inflow (*RVI*) represent an abnormal tricuspid valve. *Ao* = aorta; *LV* = left ventricle.

Fig. 15-2. Subxiphoid short-axis view of left (*LV*) ventricles shows a thick-walled RV with a small lumen. Bulging of interventricular septum into LV suggests suprasystemic RV pressure.

Fig. 15-3. Subxiphoid coronal view (L4) of right ventricular outflow tract (*RVOT*) shows narrowed infundibular area (*arrows*). RVOT is small compared with the left ventricle (*LV*). Only a portion of LV is seen from this view. *RA* = right atrium.

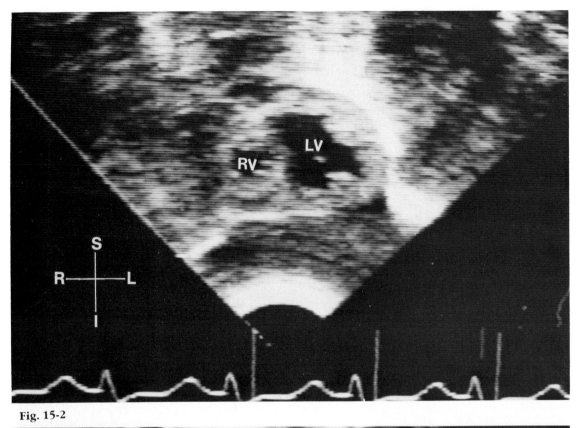

Fig. 15-2

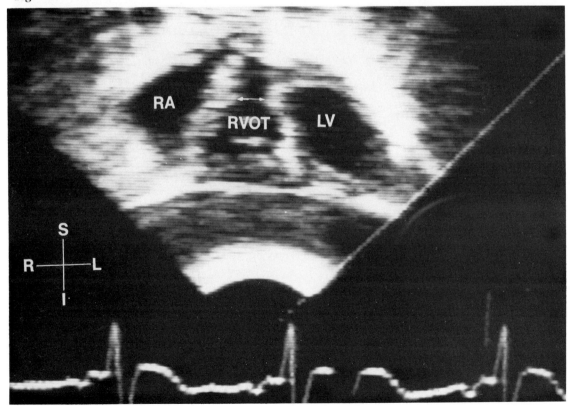

Fig. 15-3

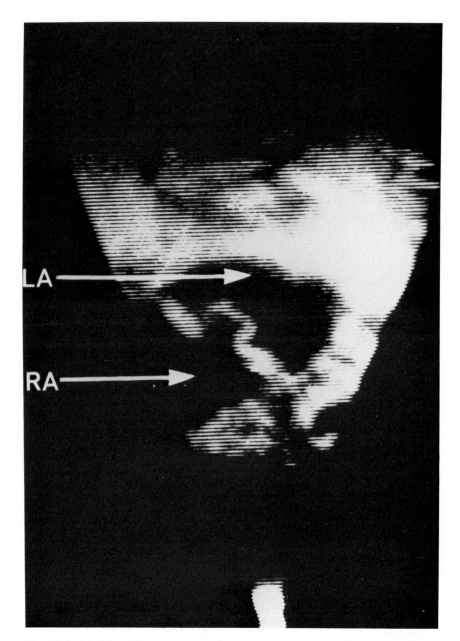

Fig. 15-4. Subxiphoid long-axis view of midatrial cavity in a patient with hypoplastic right heart. The redundant septum primum bulges into the left atrium (*LA*). Even a nonrestrictive intraatrial communication might not be demonstrated because the opening is slitlike. *RA* = right atrium.

The MPA and right and left branches of the PA (RPA and LPA, respectively) are mildly to moderately hypoplastic, as demonstrated from subxiphoid long- and short-axis, suprasternal notch (SSN), and high transverse parasternal views.

Right-to-left shunting via a patent foramen ovale is indicated by bulging of the septum primum into the left atrium (LA) throughout the cardiac cycle (Fig. 15-4). The shunt may be documented by contrast injection into a systemic vein, showing passage of contrast from RA to LA.

EXAMINATION
TECHNIQUE

The high parasternal short-axis and subxiphoid long-axis views of RV outflow (S4) best demonstrate the RV outflow, deformed pulmonary valve, and MPA. RV inflow is demonstrated in long axis from the apical 4-chamber position. Multiple sweeps in a variety of planes must be used to demonstrate the small and tortuous ductus. The best approach is to visualize the MPA–LPA junction from subxiphoid, SSN, or high-transverse positions and sweep toward the aortic arch. The presence of antegrade or retrograde flow in the MPA can be documented by Doppler examination.

PROBLEMS

The difficulties in distinguishing between the atretic and minimally patent pulmonary valve have been mentioned previously. A far more clinically important problem is the inability to assess the degree of inflow obstruction to be expected from the tricuspid valve following relief of outflow obstruction. Also the lower limit of RV size that might accommodate a normal systemic flow volume has not been established. Therefore, it is difficult to judge on the basis of echocardiographic study alone whether or not an aorticopulmonary shunt will be necessary in addition to relief of outflow obstruction.

Differentiation of pulmonary atresia with tricuspid stenosis from combined tricuspid and pulmonary atresia should not be difficult since, in the former lesion, a hypoplastic tricuspid valve forms the floor of the RA, whereas this area is usually bald in patients with tricuspid atresia.

It may be difficult to assess pulmonary blood flow by Doppler examination in hypoplastic PAs because the sample volume may be larger than the lumen of the vessel, resulting in overlap with other structures. Contrast studies may also be difficult to interpret because of small vessel size.

BIBLIOGRAPHY

Andrade, J. L., Serino, W., DeLeval, M., et al. Two-dimensional echocardiographic evaluation of tricuspid hypoplasia in pulmonary atresia. *Am. J. Cardiol.* 53: 387, 1984.

Beppu, S., Nimura, Y., and Tamai, M. Two-dimensional echocardiography in diagnosing tricuspid atresia. *Br. Heart J.* 40:1174, 1978.

Rigby, M. L., Gibson, D. G., Joseph, M. C., et al. Recognition of imperforate atrioventricular valves by two-dimensional echocardiography. *Br. Heart J.* 47:329, 1982.

Silove, E. D., DeGiovanni, J. V., Shiu, M. F., et al. Diagnosis of right ventricular outflow obstruction in infants by cross sectional echocardiography. *Br. Heart J.* 50:416, 1983.

CHAPTER 15. Hypoplastic Right Heart

Double-Chambered Right Ventricle

ANATOMY

In the *double-chambered right ventricle* (DCRV), hypertrophied muscle bundles at the margin between the right ventricular (RV) sinus and RV outflow tract obstruct RV outflow. The infundibular size is normal, and there is no displacement of the infundibular septum as in tetralogy of Fallot.

DCRV is often accompanied by a perimembranous ventricular septal defect (VSD). This defect may be small or obstructed by the muscle bundles, but when large, extends into the muscular or infundibular interventricular septum (IVS). The septal defect usually communicates with the high-pressure lower ventricular chamber and rarely with the low-pressure infundibulum. Sometimes the defect straddles the area of obstruction so that part of it communicates with the high pressure and part with the lower chamber.

Valvar pulmonary stenosis and tetralogy of Fallot are sometimes coexistent with DCRV.

Fig. 16-1. (A) Drawing of obstructive muscle bundles lying over the tricuspid valve and obstructing blood flow to the outflow tract. (B) Corresponding coronal view of right ventricle from a superiorly angulated long-axis sweep shows anomalous muscle bundles separating the right ventricular body from the infundibulum (*inf*). *LV, lv* = left ventricle; *PV* = pulmonary valve; *RA* = right atrium; *RAA* = right atrial appendage; *RV, rv* = right ventricle.

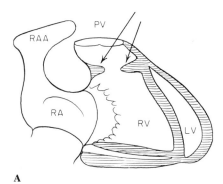

A

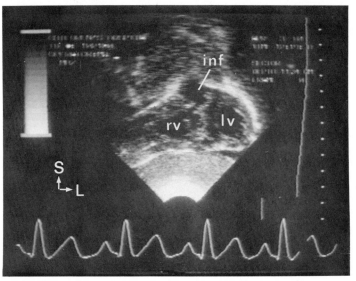

B

DIAGNOSTIC ECHO
FINDINGS

In both long- and short-axis views, muscle bundles run from the RV anterior wall to the septal band near its connection with the infundibular septum (Figs. 16-1A, B, 16-2A, B). The lumen of the RV is partially obliterated in this area.

The obstructive muscle bundles running from RV free wall to IVS may fix the midportion of the septum so that it "tents" in systole. This sensitive, but nonspecific finding alerts one to examine the RV more closely for anomalous muscle bundles.

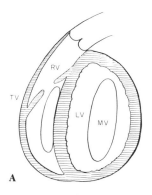

Fig. 16-2. (A) Subxiphoid short-axis view (S4) of left ventricle (*LV*) demonstrates long axis of the right ventricle (*RV*) with anomalous muscle bundles. (B) Similar echo plane demonstrates anomalous RV muscle bundles (*arrows*). *MV* = mitral valve; *TV* = tricuspid valve.

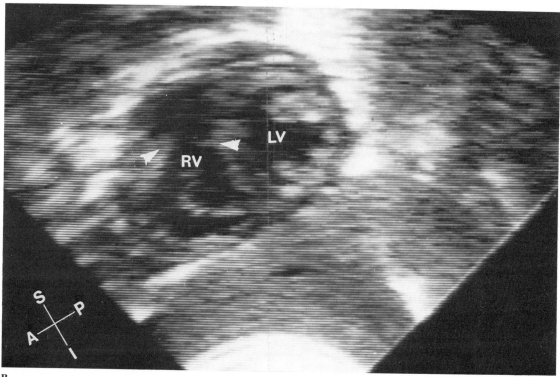

CHAPTER 16. Double-Chambered Right Ventricle

INDIRECT ECHO
FINDINGS

Supportive findings of DCRV include systolic fluttering of the pulmonary valve cusps on M-mode recording and abnormal acceleration of blood in the infundibulum by Doppler echocardiography.

ASSOCIATED LESIONS

An associated VSD will appear as dropout of echoes from the IVS, usually in the perimembranous area (see Chap. 6). The defect may be partially obscured by the overlying muscle bundles.

EXAMINATION
TECHNIQUE

Slight counterclockwise rotation of the transducer from an RV coronal plane displays the RV outflow tract in its right-left and superoinferior coordinates. The hypertrophied muscle bundles are seen encroaching upon the os infundibuli in this view. The subxiphoid short-axis (S4) view through the RV outflow tract allows assessment of the severity of narrowing in the anteroposterior (A-P) dimension.

PROBLEMS

The anomalous muscle bundles within the RV cavity are often obscured by the narrowed A-P dimension of the RV in this area. Unless there is a sufficient blood-filled cavity around the muscle bundles, they will not be visualized. The encroachment on the lumen at its midpoint may be attributed to flattening of the RV cavity and the presence of obstruction overlooked. In such cases, the supportive findings of systolic vibration pulmonary valve and increased flow velocity in the infundibular chamber by Doppler examination will direct attention to the proper diagnosis.

Clinically, DCRV may be difficult to distinguish from tetralogy of Fallot with mild RV outflow obstruction. The absence of typical findings of tetralogy of Fallot (i.e., the absence of both displacement of the infundibular septum and significant overriding of the aorta) should point toward the diagnosis of DCRV (see Chap. 27). Also, the size of the pulmonary and aortic roots are very similar in DCRV, whereas the pulmonary root is usually smaller than the aortic root in tetralogy of Fallot.

BIBLIOGRAPHY

Matina, D., Van Doesburg, N. H., Fouran, J. C., et al. Subxiphoid two-dimensional echocardiographic diagnosis of double chambered right ventricle. *Circulation* 7:885, 1983.

Riggs, T. W., Muster, A. J., Azziz, K. U., et al. Two-dimensional echocardiographic and angiocardiographic diagnosis of subpulmonary stenosis due to tricuspid valve pouch in complete transposition of the great arteries. *J. Am. Coll. Cardiol.* 1:484, 1983.

Silove, E. D., et al. Diagnosis of right ventricular outflow obstruction in infants by cross-sectional echocardiography. *Br. Heart J.* 50:416, 1983.

VonDoenhoff, L. J., and Nanda, N. C. Obstruction within the right ventricular body: Two-dimensional echocardiographic features. *Am. J. Cardiol.* 51:1498, 1983.

CHAPTER 17

Valvar Pulmonary Stenosis

ANATOMY

The stenotic pulmonary valve has fused commissures much like the stenotic aortic valve. The cusps are usually thickened. In the most severe form of dysplastic valve, the cusps resemble thick, rubbery flippers. In this form of pulmonary stenosis, the obstruction is created by the immobile, bulky cusps, not commissural fusion, and the valve does not dome in systole.

The right ventricle (RV) is usually hypertrophied, proportional to the degree of obstruction. Unless the pulmonary stenosis is critical, the volume of the RV is normal. The main and proximal left branches of the pulmonary artery (PA) are often dilated.

DIAGNOSTIC ECHO
FINDINGS

This entity is characterized by a pattern of motion as well as strictly anatomic features. Instead of moving apart against the wall of the pulmonary root, the stenotic pulmonary valve cusps dome in systole (Figs. 17-1, 17-2). During the cardiac cycle, the valve cusps move up and down as a single structure, rather than apart and together as separate cusps.

Unusual thickness of the pulmonary cusps can be demonstrated in some patients, but this finding alone is not reliable. Dilation of the main pulmonary artery (MPA) and proximal left branch is noted in older children.

Increased thickness of the RV free wall and trabeculations overlying the muscular interventricular septum (IVS) are present in patients with severe obstruction. In absolute terms, however, the wall thickness is increased only a few millimeters, limiting the sensitivity of this method in determining the presence of mild to moderate hypertrophy.

The IVS bulges toward the left ventricle (LV) during systole if RV pressure is suprasystemic.

High-velocity blood flow may be detected by Doppler sampling in the MPA, directly distal to the valve orifice.

EXAMINATION
TECHNIQUE

High transverse precordial views display the length of the RV outflow tract, pulmonary valve, and PA. A similar view from the subxiphoid short-axis position is most useful for viewing these structures in infants and small children. RV size and wall thickness may also be appreciated from the apical 4-chamber and precordial views.

Fig. 17-1. High transverse parasternal view of patient with valvar pulmonary stenosis. The pulmonary cusps dome in systole. *MPA* = main pulmonary artery; *RVOT* = right ventricular outflow tract.

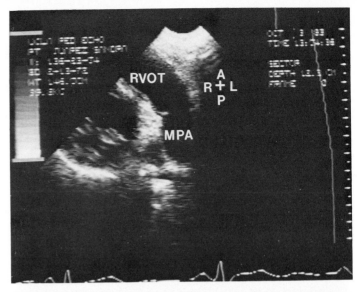

Fig. 17-2. Subxiphoid short-axis (S4) view in a young patient with moderate valvar pulmonary stenosis. The pulmonary valve (*arrow*) domes in systole. Note dilatation of the main pulmonary artery (*MPA*). *RV* = right ventricle.

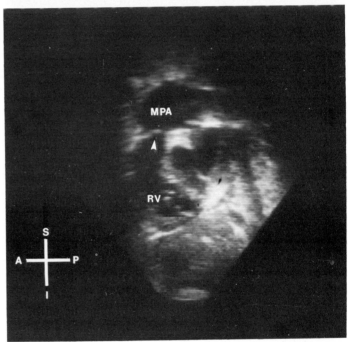

PROBLEMS

The greatest obstacle to the proper diagnosis of valvar pulmonary stenosis is poor imaging of the pulmonary valve. The high transverse precordial view usually offers a clear view of the pulmonary valve in adults and larger children unless the acoustic window is limited by lung or chest deformity. In small children and infants, the valve may be too close to this transducer position to image well: A better view is obtained from the subxiphoid short-axis views (S4).

BIBLIOGRAPHY

Weyman, A. E., Hurwitz, R. A., Girod, D. A., et al. Cross-sectional echocardiographic of visualization of the stenotic pulmonary valve. *Circulation* 56:769, 1977.

PART III. Obstructive Lesions

Congenital Mitral Obstruction

ANATOMY

This chapter covers the whole range of congenital obstruction of the mitral apparatus, from proximal to distal, since many of these lesions occur in combination (Fig. 18-1).

A supravalvar mitral ring extends centrally from the annulus into the orifice of the mitral valve. Unlike cor triatriatum, the main body of the left atrium (LA), including the fossa ovalis and left atrial appendage (LAA), is contained in the proximal, high-pressure compartment. A supravalvar mitral ring is more likely to be intimately involved with the mitral annulus and associated with other mitral abnormalities than is cor triatriatum.

In *typical congenital mitral stenosis*, the mitral leaflets and chordae tendineae may be shortened, thickened, and fused in any combination. These features are similar to the findings of rheumatic mitral stenosis.

In the *classic parachute mitral deformity*, the left ventricular (LV) papillary muscles are closely spaced and typically hypertrophied with multiple heads. Thickened chordae tendineae, converging to a single point, obstruct flow through the mitral apparatus. Rarely, two separate papillary muscles are present with only one receiving the chordal attachments. In the absence of complete atrioventricular (A-V) canal, the chordae tendineae usually converge on the posteromedial papillary muscle; in patients with complete A-V canal (septal) defect and parachute mitral deformity, the chordae tend to attach to the anterolateral papillary muscle.

These abnormalities may be found in combination with each other as well as associated with subaortic stenosis, coarctation of the aorta, ventricular septal defect (VSD), and conotruncal abnormalities.

Fig. 18-1. Composite drawing of supravalvar mitral ring with valvar stenosis and parachute deformity. The supravalvar mitral ring usually extends inward from the mitral annulus. The leaflets are foreshortened and attached to a centrally placed papillary muscle by short and fused chordae tendineae. *LV* = left ventricle; *PV* = pulmonary vein.

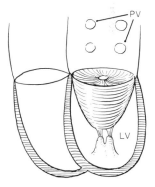

The supravalvar ring appears as a membrane bulging into the mitral valve funnel (Fig. 18-2A to C). It may be seen only in diastole when the leaflets move away from the membrane. Turbulent flow distal to the obstruction may be represented by diastolic vibrations of the mitral leaflets (M-mode) and high-velocity blood flow on Doppler examination.

Doming of the mitral valve resulting from commissural fusion of the leaflets may not be present if the leaflets are short and thick and if the obstruction is at several levels of the mitral apparatus.

The degree of thickening and foreshortening of the leaflets and chordae may be demonstrated, but cannot be related to hemodynamic abnormality.

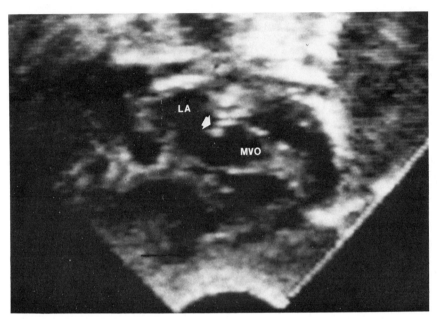

A

Fig. 18-2. (A) A subxiphoid long-axis view in a patient with supravalvar mitral ring. The membrane extends as a shelf from the mitral annulus (*arrow*). (B) This finding (*arrow*) was associated with parachute mitral valve (*mv*) and is more subtle in the parasternal long-axis view. (C) Subxiphoid 4-chamber view of a less usual type of supravalvar mitral ring shows the membrane (*arrowheads*) well into left atrium (*LA*) above the mv. Note the LA appendage (*curved arrow*) lies superior to the membrane. *AO* = aorta; *MVO* = mitral valve orifice; *RA* = right atrium.

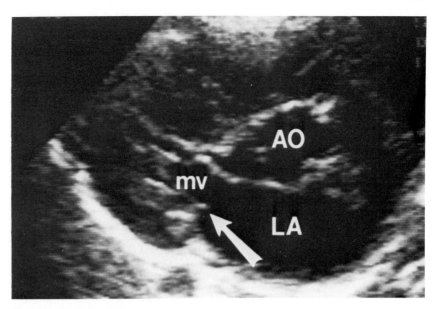

B

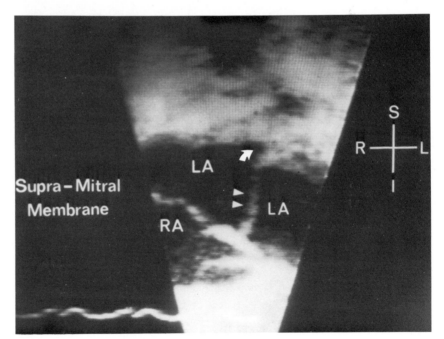

C

CHAPTER 18. Congenital Mitral Obstruction

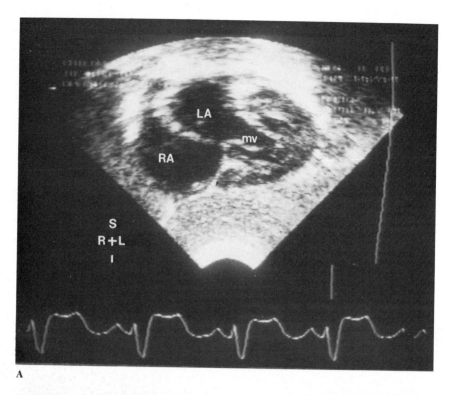

A

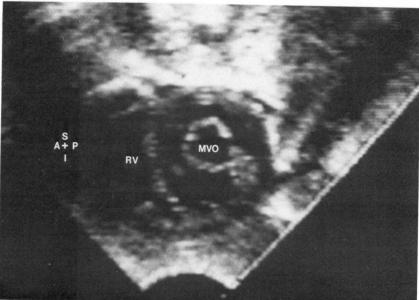

B

Fig. 18-3. (A) Subxiphoid long-axis view of left ventricle shows a centrally placed single papillary muscle. (B) Short-axis view directly above papillary muscle shows circle of chordae ten-dineae, converging on an anterolateral papillary muscle. *LA* = left atrium; *mv* = mitral valve; *MVO* = mitral valve orifice; *RA* = right atrium; *RV* = right ventricle.

PART III. Obstructive Lesions

Convergence of chordae tendineae toward a single point is characteristic of parachute mitral valve (Fig. 18-3). The valve orifice appears circular in cross section. Usually, anterior and posterior mitral leaflets cannot be separately defined.

SUPPORTIVE FINDINGS

Left atrial enlargement is present when there is significant obstruction. Findings of pulmonary hypertension may be present.

EXAMINATION TECHNIQUE

The length of the mitral valve apparatus (long axis of LV inflow tract) may be demonstrated from the precordial long-axis, apical 2- and 4-chamber, and subxiphoid 4-chamber views. These views (particularly the apical views) display a supravalvar mitral ring, doming of the mitral valve, and the length of the mitral leaflets and chordae tendineae. The usual type of supravalvar mitral ring is only visualized in diastole, when the mitral leaflets move away from the membrane. To display the characteristics of parachute mitral valve, the transducer is turned to a LV short-axis plane (left parasternal or subxiphoid position) and swept from mitral leaflet to the papillary muscles.

PROBLEMS

It is difficult to determine the most significant area of obstruction when there are multiple mitral abnormalities.

There are no criteria to determine the presence or severity of obstruction in parachute mitral valve.

In the presence of severe LV outflow obstruction or ventricular dysfunction, cardiac output may be so low that the mitral valve does not open fully, masking the findings of congenital mitral stenosis or supravalvar mitral ring.

The absence of doming may mask obstruction of the mitral leaflets.

BIBLIOGRAPHY

Driscoll, D. J., Gutgesell, H. P., and McNamara, D. G. Echocardiographic features of congenital mitral stenosis. *Am. J. Cardiol.* 42:259, 1978.

Gutgessel, H. P., Cheatham, J., Latson, L. A., et al. Atrioventricular valve abnormalities in infancy: Two-dimensional echocardiographic and angiocardiographic comparison. *J. Am. Coll. Cardiol.* 2:531, 1983.

Jacobstein, M. D., and Hirschfeld, S. S. Concealed left atrial membrane: Pitfalls in the diagnosis of cor triatriatum and supravalve mitral ring. *Am. J. Cardiol.* 49: 780, 1982.

Layman, T. E., and Edwards, J. E. Anomalous mitral arcade: A type of congenital mitral insufficiency. *Circulation* 35:389, 1967.

Parr, G. V. S., Fripp, R. R., Whitman, V., et al. Anomalous mitral arcade: Echocardiographic and angiographic recognition. *Pediatr. Cardiol.* 4:163, 1983.

Snider, A. R., Roger, L. L., Schiller, M. B., and Silverman, N. H. Congenital left ventricular inflow obstruction evaluated by two-dimensional echocardiography. *Circulation* 61:4:848, 1980.

CHAPTER 18. Congenital Mitral Obstruction

Cor Triatriatum

ANATOMY

A membrane with a variably sized opening separates the proximal left atrial (LA) chamber, which receives the pulmonary veins (PVs), from the distal chamber, which includes the fossa ovalis, atrial appendage, and mitral annulus. The PVs and proximal chamber are dilated if the membrane is obstructive. The membrane lies obliquely across the LA, extending inferiorly and posteriorly from a superior and anterior location behind the aortic root. In older patients, the membrane may be calcified. The mitral apparatus is usually normal.

Long-standing PV hypertension may lead to pulmonary artery (PA) hypertension and finally to right ventricular (RV) hypertrophy and dilation.

DIAGNOSTIC ECHO
FINDINGS

A curved membrane lies across the LA, dividing it into a proximal portion receiving the PVs and a distal portion containing fossa ovalis and left atrial appendage (LAA) (Fig. 19-1). These features distinguish cor triatriatum from supravalvar mitral ring, in which the fossa ovalis and LAA are related to the proximal chamber.

The PVs and proximal atrial chamber are dilated when there is significant obstruction; the membrane bulges downward toward the mitral annulus.

Diastolic fluttering of the mitral leaflets and high-velocity flow (by Doppler examination) in the distal atrial chamber and mitral orifice are present.

Abnormal RV systolic time intervals, RV hypertrophy, and RV dilation, if present, indicate secondary PA hypertension.

The mitral valve is usually normal.

Fig. 19-1. Drawing shows the usual relationship of the membrane of cor triatriatum with the foramen ovale, left atrial appendage, and mitral annulus. *LA* = left atrium; *LV* = left ventricle; *RA* = right atrium; *RV* = right ventricle.

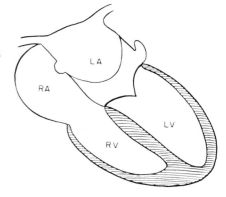

EXAMINATION
TECHNIQUE

The apical and subxiphoid 4-chamber views (Fig. 19-2) display the LA from PVs to mitral annulus and therefore demonstrate the obstructive membrane. These views may also show the fossa ovalis related to the distal atrial chamber. The precordial long-axis and apical 2-chamber views display the membrane and details of the mitral valve apparatus.

PROBLEMS

Patients with cor triatriatum are frequently sent to the noninvasive laboratory with a clinical diagnosis of valvar mitral stenosis. Fortunately, these lesions can be easily distinguished from each other. Differentiating cor triatriatum from supravalvar mitral ring may be more difficult because of the need to demonstrate the relationship of the membrane to the LAA and fossa ovalis. Occasionally, the obstructing membrane may lie across or below the foramen ovale, making the differential diagnosis with supravalvar mitral ring very difficult. However, the latter is usually more intimately involved with the mitral annulus. Operationally, it is more important to note whether there is an associated mitral valve anomaly.

The obstructing membrane may be difficult to visualize because its extreme curvature deflects some echoes out of the returning beam path.

Fig. 19-2. Apical 4-chamber of patient with cor triatriatum. The membrane lies across the left atrium between the mitral annulus and the lower left pulmonary vein (*LPV*). High-velocity flow distal to this membrane is demonstrated by the Doppler signal on the left. *AN* = mitral annulus; *LA* = left atrium; *M* = membrane; *RA* = right atrium.

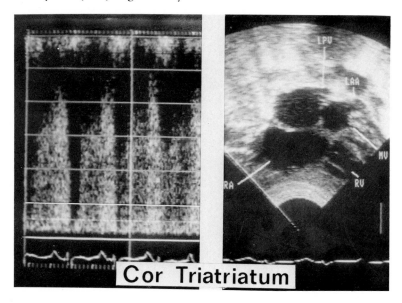

Cor Triatriatum

CHAPTER 19. Cor Triatriatum

BIBLIOGRAPHY

Jacobstein, M. D., and Hirschfeld, S. S. Concealed left atrial membrane: Pitfalls in the diagnosis of cortriatriatum and supravalve mitral ring. *Am. J. Cardiol.* 49:780, 1982.

Marin-Garcia, J., Amplatz, K., Moiler, J. H., et al. Cortriatriatum and atrial septal defect. *Am. Heart J.* 87:238, 1974.

Marin-Garcia, J., Tandon, R., Lucas, R. V., et al. Cortriatriatum: Study of 20 cases. *Am. J. Cardiol.* 35:59, 1975.

Norell, M. S., Lincoln, C., and Sutton, G. C. Two-dimensional echocardiographic diagnosis of cor triatriatum. *J. Cardiovasc. Ultrasonogr.* 2:369, 1983.

Schluter, M., Lagenstein, B. A., Thier, W., et al. Transesophageal two-dimensional echocardiography in the diagnosis of cortriatriatum in the adult. *J. Am. Coll. Cardiol.* 2:1011, 1983.

Snider, A. R., Roge, C. L., Schiller, N. B., et al. Congenital left ventricular inflow obstruction evaluated by two-dimensional echocardiography. *Circulation* 61:848, 1978.

Weindorf, S., Goldberg, H., Goldman, M., et al. Diagnosis of cortriatriatum by two-dimensional echocardiography. *J. Clin. Ultrasound* 9:97, 1981.

Hypoplastic Left Heart Syndrome: Mitral and Aortic Atresia

ANATOMY

The classic description of *hypoplastic left heart syndrome* includes hypoplasia of the left heart (i.e., atrium, mitral valve, left ventricle [LV], and ascending aorta), in addition to atresia of the aortic valve (Fig. 20-1). Pulmonary venous (PV) blood must exit the left atrium (LA) via a patent foramen ovale or atrial septal defect (ASD). The mitral valve may be an imperforate membrane, stenotic or small, but perfectly formed. The LV is only a few millimeters in diameter unless mitral regurgitation or a ventricular septal defect (VSD) allows blood flow through the chamber. In rare circumstances, this blood flow is sufficient to provide near-normal growth of the ventricle.

The aortic valve is a small gelatinous mass at the base of the aortic root. The ascending aorta only receives retrograde bloodflow from the descending aorta via a patent ductus arteriosus (PDA) and is approximately the size of the coronary arteries it supplies. Discrete coarctation of the aorta may be present in addition to tubular hypoplasia of the transverse arch. A large PDA supplies a normal-sized descending aorta (Fig. 20-2). The right ventricle (RV) and pulmonary arteries (PAs) are dilated.

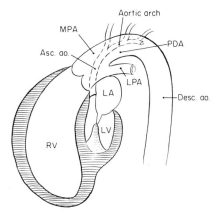

Fig. 20-1. Diagram of aortic atresia with hypoplastic left ventricle (*LV*) as seen from the left side. The diminutive LV contains a proportionally smaller mitral valve, here shown as a parachute valve. The LV long axis is foreshortened and does not reach the cardiac apex. The aortic root is small and contains nonmoving echoes of an imperforate aortic valve. The dilated and hypertrophied right ventricle (*RV*) gives rise to the main pulmonary artery (*MPA*), which forms an arch by its continuity with the descending aorta (*Desc. ao.*) via a patent ductus arteriosus (*PDA*). The ascending aorta (*Asc. ao.*) lies to the right of the MPA; the aortic arch lies to the right of the ductus arteriosus. *LA* = left atrium; *LPA* = left pulmonary artery.

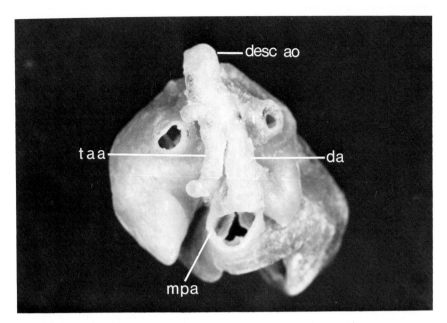

Fig. 20-2. View from the top of a fixed perfused heart of a patient with aortic atresia showing the ductus arteriosus (*da*) and transverse aortic arch (*taa*) lying side by side. Note the brachio- cephalic vessels arising from the aortic arch. The main pulmonary artery (*mpa*) has been opened to show the pulmonary valve. *desc ao* = descending aorta.

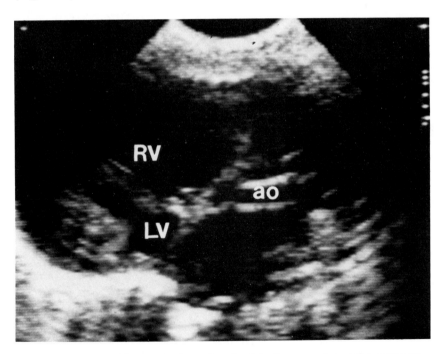

Fig. 20-3. Parasternal long-axis view of an atretic aortic valve and ascending aorta. The ascending aorta is approx- imately the same size as the coronary arteries. *ao* = aortic root; *LV* = left ventricle; *RV* = right ventricle.

PART III. Obstructive Lesions

DIAGNOSTIC ECHO
FINDINGS

Nonmoving echoes from the aortic valve primordium are located within a
hypoplastic aortic root (Fig. 20-3). The coronary arteries rise from the small
ascending aorta. The ascending aorta is the size of the coronary arteries or
slightly larger. No antegrade flow is registered in the ascending aorta by
Doppler studies, but often the sample volume overlaps the nearby PA or superior vena cava (SVC) so that an unambiguous signal cannot be obtained.

The LV long axis does not reach the cardiac apex, which is formed by the
RV. The short-axis diameter is also smaller than normal, ranging from a
minuscule slit to up to 1 cm (Fig. 20-4A to C).

Fig. 20-4. Subxiphoid long-axis view of
left ventricular outflow in a normal
heart (A) and hypoplastic left ventricle
(*LV*) (B). The long axis of the hypoplastic *LV* is foreshortened and does not
reach the cardiac apex. Subxiphoid
short-axis view of hypoplastic *LV* (C),
which has a small lumen and thick
walls. The long axis of the right ventricle (*RV*) and outflow tract (*RVOT*) is
displayed. *PV* = pulmonary valve;
RA = right atrium.

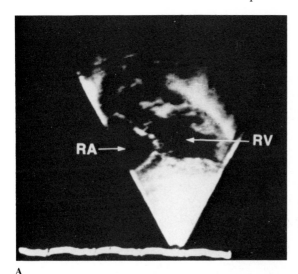

A

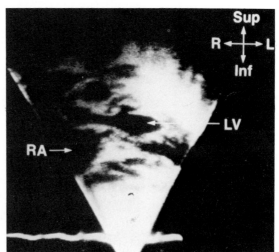

B

C

The mitral valve's appearance is often nondescript because the LV is too small for adequate display of the subvalvar apparatus (Fig. 20-5). The motion of even an imperforate membrane may simulate valve-opening. Doppler echocardiography can be used to determine the presence or absence of ventricular inflow if the ventricle is large enough to contain the sample volume without overlap of other structures.

The floor of the LA, the area of the mitral annulus, is small. In patients with increased PV return, the septum primum bulges into the right atrium (RA) unless there is decompression via a large interatrial septal defect (Fig. 20-6).

A PDA connects the main pulmonary artery (MPA) and descending aorta, forming an arch (Fig. 20-7). Partial constriction of the ductus may be seen at its aortic end. The response of the ductus arteriosus to pharmacologic intervention may be followed by serial studies.

Fig. 20-5. Subxiphoid 4-chamber view of a patient with aortic atresia shows a normally formed but hypoplastic mitral valve within a diminutive left ventricle. *LA* = left atrium; *RA* = right atrium.

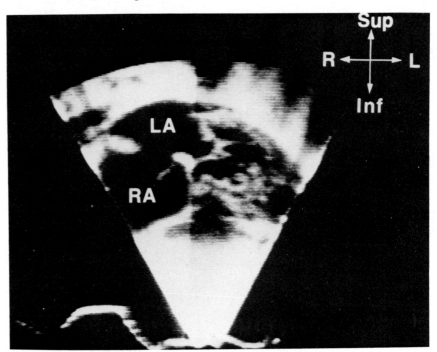

Fig. 20-7. Subxiphoid long-axis view of the right ventricle (*RV*) shows arch formed by main pulmonary artery (*MPA*), patent ductus arteriosus (*PDA*), and descending aorta (*Desc Ao*). *PV* = pulmonary valve.

PART III. Obstructive Lesions

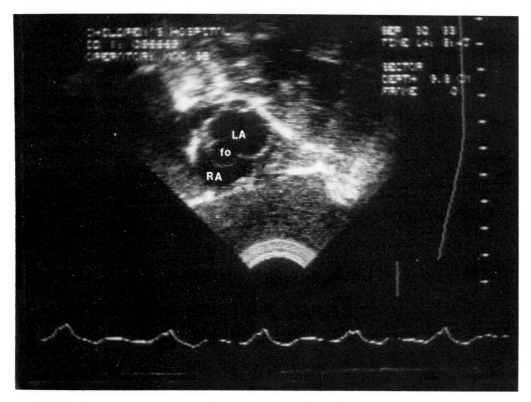

Fig. 20-6. Subxiphoid short-axis view of atria shows foramen ovale (*fo*) with restrictive septum primum bulging into the right atrium (*RA*) to provide outflow from the left atrium (*LA*) in a patient with aortic atresia.

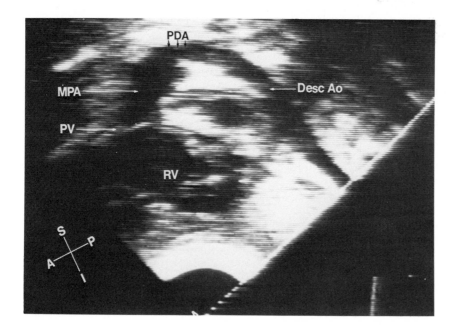

CHAPTER 20. Hypoplastic Left Heart Syndrome: Mitral and Aortic Atresia

The RV and PAs are dilated and appear strikingly so in comparison with the hypoplastic left heart structures.

EXAMINATION
TECHNIQUE

The subxiphoid and precordial views are useful in defining all segments of the left heart: LV inflow tract by subxiphoid and apical 4-chamber views, LV outflow tract by subxiphoid and parasternal long-axis views, and so on. Excellent lateral and axial resolution is required to demonstrate these very small structures. The LV may appear at first as a recess in the posterior RV wall. It is helpful to identify the interatrial septum first, then the mitral valve to its left (see Fig. 20-3). In doing so, the LV inflow tract is displayed. The aorta may be identified by careful scanning to the right of the dilated MPA in a subxiphoid suprasternal notch (SSN) or left parasternal long-axis plane. The aortic arch appears to the right of the ductus arteriosus and may be identified by the brachiocephalic vessels rising from it.

VARIATIONS

If a large interventricular communication or mitral regurgitation exists, the LV may approach normal size in short axis, but usually does not reach the cardiac apex in long-axis views.

Coarctation of the aorta, if present, is difficult to ascertain because of the small size of the transverse aortic arch and the close proximity of the PDA to the distal arch.

PROBLEMS

Aortic atresia cannot be diagnosed unless the hypoplastic ascending aorta and its origin are clearly demonstrated. The arch formed by MPA, large PDA, and descending aorta may superficially resemble an aortic arch rising from the RV until one notes that (1) PA branches rise laterally from the ascending portion (seen on other views) and (2) there are no brachiocephalic branches rising from the arch-forming segment, the PDA.

As mentioned previously, an associated coarctation of the aorta cannot be confidently excluded due to the small lumen of the distal transverse arch and its proximity to the ductus.

BIBLIOGRAPHY

Lange, L. W., Sahn, D. J., Allen, H. D., et al. Cross-sectional echocardiography in hypoplastic left ventricle: Echocardiographic, angiographic, anatomic correlations. *Pediatr. Cardiol.* 1:287, 1980.

Rigby, M. L., Gibson, D. G., Joseph, M. C., et al. Recognition of imperforate atrioventricular valves by two-dimensional echocardiography. *Br. Heart J.* 47:329, 1982.

Fixed Left Ventricular Outflow Obstruction

ANATOMY

Fixed left ventricular (LV) outflow obstruction may take the form of a discrete membrane or fibromuscular ridge beneath the aortic cusps or a long tunnellike muscular obstruction of the LV outflow tract (Fig. 21-1A to C). In discrete or short-segment obstruction, the proximal or midportion of the anterior mitral leaflet may be tethered or pulled toward the interventricular septum (IVS) by the membrane. In one form of long-segment obstruction, a muscular cuff separates the anterior mitral annulus from the aortic annulus, creating discontinuity between these fibrous structures. In another form of long-segment obstruction, the infundibular septum is displaced posteriorly, encroaching on the LV outflow tract. This latter form is usually associated with a malalignment-type ventricular septal defect (VSD) and may be associated with normally related or transposed great arteries (TGA).

In most cases of discrete fixed obstruction, a jet of blood is directed toward one or two cusps of the semilunar valve. The cusps may be thickened and regurgitant as a result of this turbulence. The aortic valve may also be intrinsically abnormal and stenotic.

LV hypertrophy may be present, depending on the severity of obstruction. Poststenotic dilation of the ascending aorta is relatively uncommon but can occur.

Fig. 21-1. Three different types of subaortic stenosis. (A) A discrete subaortic ring attaching the anterior mitral leaflet to the left septal surface. The mitral leaflet may be pulled toward the septum as shown here. (B) Long-segment, tunnel-type subaortic stenosis with muscle encircling the left ventricular outflow tract, encroaching on the lumen and creating discontinuity between the mitral and aortic annuli. (C) Subaortic stenosis caused by posterior displacement of the infundibular septum. *Ao* = aortic root; *LA* = left atrium; *LV* = left ventricle; *RV* = right ventricle.

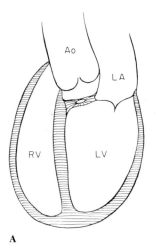
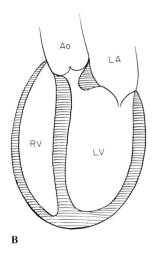
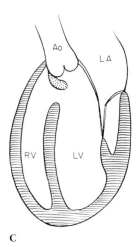

A   B   C

A thin subaortic membrane may sometimes be visualized from the left parasternal or subxiphoid long-axis views (Fig. 21-2), but is more clearly demonstrated from the apical 2-chamber view (Fig. 21-3). With fibromuscular obstruction, there may be a wedge-shaped muscular base extending from the IVS. Depending on whether the muscular component projects from the anterior or medial aspect of the septal border of the outflow tract, it may be better visualized from the parasternal or subxiphoid long-axis views, respectively.

Long-segment obstruction appears as a narrowed muscular channel beneath the aortic valve. In such cases, the aortic valve may be displaced superiorly. If posterior deviation of the outflow (infundibular) septum is responsible for the obstruction, this structure, malaligned from the lower muscular septum, encroaches upon the anterior aspect of the LV outflow tract (Fig. 21-4). This displacement, usually associated with a malalignment VSD, is best viewed from the parasternal long-axis and subxiphoid short-axis views showing the A-P position of the infundibular septum.

Fig. 21-2. Parasternal long-axis view of discrete fibrous subaortic stenosis. A redundant ring of fibrous tissue (*arrow*) lies across the outflow tract and is attached to the left septal surface and anterior mitral leaflet. Note the thick muscular base on the septal side of the membrane. *AO* = aortic root; *LA* = left atrium; *LV* = left ventricle.

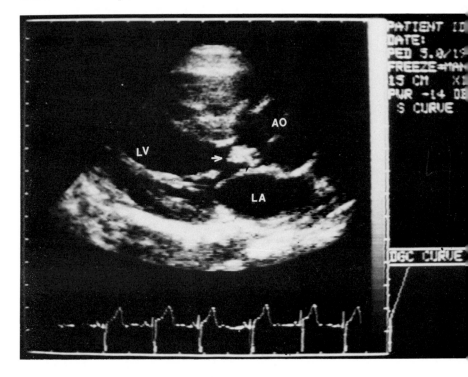

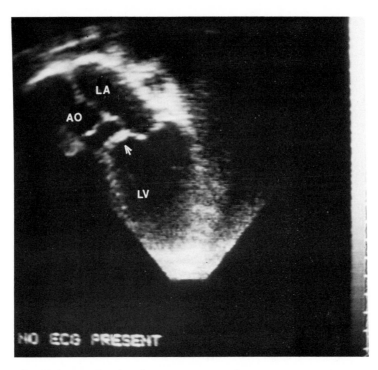

Fig. 21-3. Apical 2-chamber view in discrete subaortic stenosis. The membrane (*arrow*) is seen 1 cm beneath the aortic cusps. *AO* = aortic root; *LA* = left atrium; *LV* = left ventricle.

Fig. 21-4. Parasternal long-axis view of patient with a posteriorly malaligned infundibular septum (*arrow*), causing subpulmonary stenosis in a patient with transposition of the great arteries. Note the small pulmonary root. This is similar in appearance to a malalignment type of subaortic obstruction in normally related great arteries. *LA* = left atrium; *LV* = left ventricle; *PA* = pulmonary artery; *RV* = right ventricle. (The authors thank Dr. Lennis Burke for this illustration.)

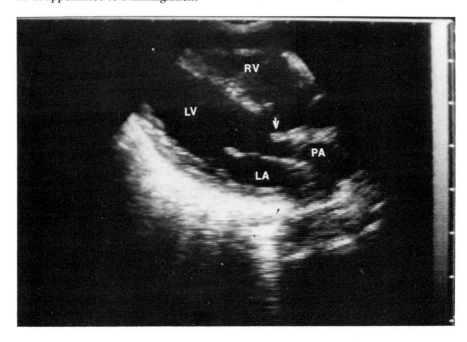

INDIRECT FINDINGS

Coarse fluttering of the aortic valve (or pulmonary valve in TGA) during systole is a sensitive finding and often the first indication of outflow obstruction. In fixed subaortic stenosis, the jet usually strikes only one or two cusps, causing systolic flutter and partial closure while the other cusps move normally. In dynamic outflow obstruction, all cusps show early-midsystolic closure, reflecting a change in flow dynamics.

LV hypertrophy may be present. With significant obstruction, the ratio of end-systolic wall thickness to short-axis dimension may be increased as a nonspecific indication of pressure overload.

Systolic anterior motion of the anterior mitral leaflet on M-mode recording is an uncommon finding in fixed or discrete subaortic stenosis. When present, the configuration is peaked, rather than flattopped as in obstructive hypertrophic cardiomyopathy. Its cause and implications are not agreed on, but are probably related to a Venturi effect caused by high-velocity bloodflow at the point of obstruction, the peak of anterior motion occurring at peak ejection velocity.

EXAMINATION TECHNIQUE

Parasternal long-axis and apical 2-chamber views display the anteroposterior (A-P) coordinates of the LV outflow tract; the subxiphoid long-axis view displays the right-left coordinates of that area. The apical 2-chamber view best displays a fibrous subaortic membrane because the echo beam is perpendicular to the weakly reflective membrane. Short-axis sweeps from the left parasternal and subxiphoid positions yield cross-sections of the outflow tract. Long-axis views are better for defining the exact position and type of LV outflow obstruction; short-axis views may display the cross-sectional area of the lumen at the site of obstruction.

PROBLEMS

The greatest problem with diagnosing membranous subaortic stenosis is the aforementioned difficulty in visualizing the weakly reflective membrane. The presence of systolic fluttering of the aortic cusps should prompt an intensive exploration of the LV ouflow tract, with special attention given to obtaining a good quality apical 2-chamber view. Doppler sampling proximal to the aortic valve will show increased flow velocity and help to distinguish between valvular and subvalvular subaortic stenosis. Manipulation of gain and display settings will facilitate recording of these weak echoes.

In fibromuscular obstruction, it is helpful for the surgeon to know the inferior extent of the muscular base, since this is poorly visualized in the usual operative approach from the aorta. In some cases, the IVS may be pulled into the outflow tract by traction from a subaortic membrane, but the septum is not actually thickened at that point, making aggressive resection more likely to result in an interventricular septal defect. Careful measurement of septal thickness with good visualization of the right as well as left septal thickness is required in order to assess the need for and extent of surgical resection.

It is possible for fixed, short-segment obstruction to coexist with typical hypertrophic cardiomyopathy. Examination of the LV outflow tract from all available views should disclose this rare association.

PART III. Obstructive Lesions

As yet, neither wall thickness nor cross-sectional area of the outflow tract has been directly related to pressure gradient in discrete subaortic stenosis; however, severe obstruction results in obvious alterations in these parameters. Doppler echocardiography has proved invaluable for estimation of gradient by peak flow velocity and determining the site and severity of obstruction.

When fixed LV ouflow obstruction is present in D-TGA, the LV outflow tract is so compressed that an obstructing membrane may not be visualized. Also, a bright echo on the left septal surface, resulting from contact with the anterior mitral leaflet, may simulate a structure within the outflow tract.

BIBLIOGRAPHY

Berry, T. E., Aziz, K. U., and Paul, M. H. Echocardiographic assessment of discrete subaortic stenosis in childhood. *Am. J. Cardiol.* 43:957, 1979.

Brenner, J. I., Baker, K., Ringel, R. E., et al. Echocardiographic evidence of left ventricular bands in infants and children. *J. Am. Coll. Cardiol.* 3:1515, 1984.

Chung, K. J., Fulton, D. R., Kriedberg, M. B., et al. Combined discrete subaortic stenosis and ventricular septal defect in infants and children. *Am. J. Cardiol.* 53:1429, 1984.

Del Guzzo, L., and Sherrid, M. V. Anomalous papillary muscle insertion contributing to obstruction in discrete subaortic stenosis. *J. Am. Coll. Cardiol.* 2:379, 1983.

Di Sessa, T. G., Hagen, A. D., Isabel-Jones, J. B., et al. Two-dimensional echocardiographic evaluation of discrete subaortic stenosis from the apical long axis view. *Am. Heart J.* 101:774, 1981.

Ebels, T., Meijboom, E. J., Anderson, R. H., et al. Anatomic and functional "obstruction" of the outflow tract in atrioventricular septal defects with separate valve orifices ("ostium primum atrial septal defect"): An echocardiographic study. *Am. J. Cardiol.* 54:843, 1984.

Freedom, R. M., Dische, M. R., and Rowe, R. D. Pathologic anatomy of subaortic stenosis and atresia in the first year of life. *Am. J. Cardiol.* 39:1035, 1977.

Gow, R. M., Freedom, R. M., Williams, W. G., et al. Coarctation of the aorta or subaortic stenosis with atrioventricular septal defect. *Am. J. Cardiol.* 53:1421, 1984.

Kreuger, S. K., French, J. W., Forker, A. D., et al. Echocardiography in discrete subaortic stenosis. *Circulation* 59:506, 1979.

Lappen, R. S., Muster, A. J., Idriss, F. S., et al. Masked subaortic stenosis in ostium primum atrial septal defect: Recognition and treatment. *Am. J. Cardiol.* 52:336, 1983.

Nishimura, T., Kondo, M., Umadome, H., et al. Echocardiographic features of false tendons in the left ventricle. *Am. J. Cardiol.* 48:177, 1981.

Perry, L. W., Ruckman, R. N., Shapiro, S. R., et al. Left ventricular false tendons in children: Prevalence as detected by 2-dimensional echocardiography and clinical significance. *Am. J. Cardiol.* 52:1264, 1983.

Rutkowski, M., Damlowiez, D., Doyle, E. F., et al. An unusual type of discrete subvalvar aortic stenosis, demonstrated by two-dimensional echocardiography. *J. Cardiovasc. Ultrasonogr.* 3:283, 1982.

Wenink, A. C. G., and Gittenberger-de Groot, A. C. Straddling mitral and tricuspid valves: Morphologic differences and developmental backgrounds. *Am. J. Cardiol.* 49:1959, 1982.

Wilcox, W. D., Seward, J. B., Hagler, D. J., et al. Discrete subaortic stenosis: Two-dimensional features with angiographic and surgical correlation. *Mayo Clin. Proc.* 55:425, 1980.

Williams, D. E., Sahn, D. J., and Friedman, W. F. Cross-sectional echocardiographic localization of sites of left ventricular outflow tract obstruction. *Am. J. Cardiol.* 37:250, 1976.

CHAPTER 21. Fixed Left Ventricular Outflow Obstruction

Hypertrophic Cardiomyopathy

ANATOMY

The most commonly recognized form of familial hypertrophic cardiomyopathy involves a remarkable focal thickening of the upper subaortic region of the interventricular septum (IVS). The remainder of the septum and left ventricular (LV) free wall may also be hypertrophied to a lesser and more uniform degree. The LV is banana-shaped. The ventricular cavity is often obliterated in systole at the level of the papillary muscles. The tips of the mitral leaflets are pulled into close apposition to the IVS. In addition, the midportion of the anterior mitral leaflet may be drawn into the LV outflow tract by decreased lateral pressure caused by increased flow velocity (i.e., Venturi effect). Although there is continuing debate about the usual site of outflow obstruction, whether at midleaflet, leaflet edge, or papillary muscles, it is safe to say that obstruction has been observed at all these locations in some patients.

Important anatomic variations of this disease include severe symmetric hypertrophy as well as focal hypertrophy of the lower muscular septum, papillary muscles, or LV free wall.

The gross anatomic appearance of the heart in hypertrophic cardiomyopathy, which is found in infants of diabetic mothers, is similar to severe symmetric or focal hypertrophy, except there may be a uniform thickening of the right ventricular (RV) and LV free walls, with only mild to moderate asymmetric hypertrophy of the IVS.

DIAGNOSTIC ECHO
FINDINGS

Asymmetric hypertrophy of the upper portion of the IVS is best demonstrated from parasternal and apical (2-chamber) long-axis views (Fig. 22-1A). Other areas of thickening of the inflow septum or LV free wall are best displayed by short-axis sweeps from the left parasternal border or subxiphoid positions (Figs. 22-1B, 22-2). The involved segments show poor wall motion and diminished systolic thickening. In addition, fibrosis within the myocardium may give it a speckled appearance. The subxiphoid long-axis (L3) view displays a more medial portion of the septum, which may also be involved (Fig. 22-3).

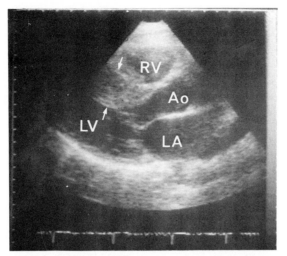

A

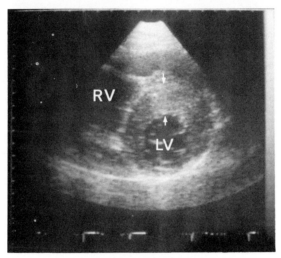

B

Fig. 22-1. Parasternal long-axis (A) and short-axis (B) views of left ventricle (*LV*) in a patient with hypertrophic obstructive cardiomyopathy. The upper portion of the interventricular septum (*arrows*) is thickened. *Ao* = aortic root; *LA* = left atrium; *RV* = right ventricle.

CHAPTER 22. Hypertrophic Cardiomyopathy

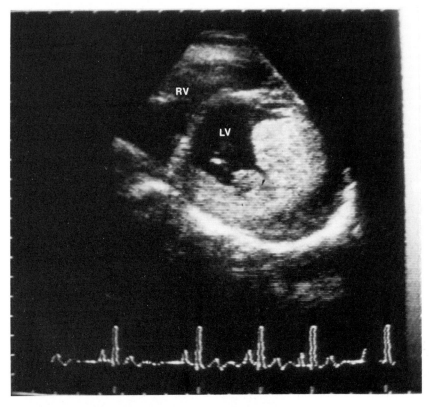

Fig. 22-2. Parasternal short-axis view at the level of the papillary muscles in a patient with hypertrophic cardiomyopathy involving only the papillary muscles and free wall. Note the normal thickness of the interventricular septum. This patient had poor diastolic compliance but no outflow obstruction. *LV* = left ventricle; *RV* = right ventricle.

Fig. 22-3. Subxiphoid long-axis view of left ventricular outflow in a patient with multiple rhabdomyomas, involving right and left ventricles (*lv*). Note that the tumors (*arrows*) have a distinct echo-dense appearance compared with normal myocardium. *ao* = aortic root; *ra* = right atrium.

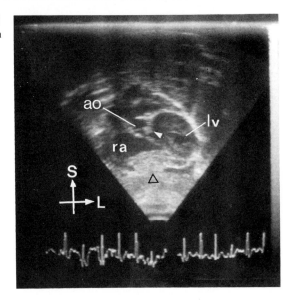

PART III. Obstructive Lesions

INDIRECT FINDINGS

The following findings suggest dynamic left ventricular outflow obstruction: (1) fluttering and midsystolic closure of all aortic leaflets (compared with flutter of only one leaflet in discrete or fixed subaortic stenosis); (2) systolic anterior motion of the mid- or distal portion of the anterior mitral leaflet toward the IVS (this motion characteristically occurs during midsystole, the valve returning to a normal position before the end of systole); (3) anacrotic shoulder on carotid-pulse tracing temporally associated with an ejection murmur (the ejection time may be prolonged, while the early systolic upstroke [T ½] is normal); and (4) Doppler flow patterns at or slightly below the aortic valve may show high-velocity flow with cessation of flow in midsystole, depending on the severity of obstruction.

EXAMINATION
TECHNIQUE

All available views must be used to image the entire IVS and the RV and LV free walls. It is important to image the long axis of the LV outflow tract from the parasternal, apical, and subxiphoid long-axis views. The precordial views show the most common sites of obstruction between the IVS and the mid- and distal portions of the anterior mitral leaflet. The subxiphoid long-axis view demonstrates rare variations in which there may be attachments of the mitral valve to the septum or other accessory mitral tissue.

The anatomic information provided by two-dimensional studies is complemented by physiologic data supplied by M-mode recordings, carotid-pulse recordings, and phonocardiography. Ideally, the M-mode recording is directed from the two-dimensional images. These studies may be performed at rest and with provocative maneuvers such as Valsalva, standing, and squatting as well as inhalation of amyl nitrate (use with caution and only in individuals with no demonstrable obstruction at rest) in order to profile the nature of obstruction under a variety of physiologic conditions.

PROBLEMS

It is usually easy to diagnose the presence of hypertrophic cardiomyopathy; evaluation of the severity of outflow tract obstruction may be more difficult. Nevertheless, characterization of outflow obstruction by the maneuvers described previously may give relevant information about the presence of a gradient during daily activities. Obviously, serial studies provide invaluable data concerning response to therapy.

Very rarely, typical hypertrophic cardiomyopathy is associated with fixed as well as dynamic obstruction.

Infiltrative cardiomyopathy may cause symmetric or focal thickening of the myocardium, similar to hypertrophic cardiomyopathy. In general, however, wall motion and systolic thickening are more impaired and the density of myocardium more altered with infiltrative than with hypertrophic disease.

Rhabdomyomas appear as single or multiple focal masses within the myocardium and are easily distinguished from hypertrophic cardiomyopathy by their echo-dense appearance, quite different from normal or even fibrotic myocardium (Fig. 22-3).

CHAPTER 22. Hypertrophic Cardiomyopathy

BIBLIOGRAPHY

Gutgesell, H. T., Spear, M. D., and Rosenberg, H. Characterization of the cardiomyopathy in infants of diabetic mothers. *Circulation* 61:441, 1980.

Maron, B. J., Gottdiener, J. S., Bonow, R. O., and Epstein, S. E. Hypertrophic cardiomyopathy with unusual location of left ventricular hypertrophy undetectable by M-mode echocardiographic identification by wide angle two dimensional echocardiography. *Circulation* 63:409, 1981.

Marx, G. R., Bierman, F. Z., Matthews, E., et al. Two-dimensional echocardiographic diagnosis of intracardiac masses in infancy. *J. Am. Coll. Cardiol.* 3:827, 1984.

Ports, T. A., Cogan, J., Schiller, N. B., et al. Echocardiography of left ventricular masses. *Circulation* 58:528, 1978.

Shapiro, L. M., and McKenna, W. J. Distribution of left ventricular hypertrophy in hypertrophic cardiomyopathy: A two-dimensional echocardiographic study. *J. Am. Coll. Cardiol.* 52:544, 1983.

PART III. Obstructive Lesions

Valvar Aortic Stenosis

ANATOMY

The stenotic aortic valve is commonly bicommissural, with one large cusp containing a raphe (underdeveloped commissure) and a small cusp. The resulting line of coaptation is eccentric within the aortic root. More rarely, the stenotic valve is tricommissural with partial fusion of the commissures. Like the bicommissural valve, the tricommissural valve orifice may be eccentric. The abnormal thickness and irregular margins of the stenotic valve create a redundant closure line in diastole. Infants with critical aortic stenosis frequently have a thick, myxomatous, unicommissural valve with an eccentric, pinhole orifice.

The proximal ascending aorta is often dilated in children and adults with aortic stenosis, but hypoplastic to some degree in infants with critical aortic stenosis.

Most children and young adults with aortic stenosis have an appropriate degree of left ventricular (LV) hypertrophy, which allows compensation for the pressure overload. The increase in LV mass is roughly proportional to the severity of the aortic stenosis. Systolic function parameters are usually normal or hyperdynamic. In contrast, the LV of infants with critical aortic stenosis may have a large lumen, thin wall, and poor systolic contraction or a small lumen and thick wall with endocardial fibroelastosis.

DIAGNOSTIC ECHO FINDINGS

Systolic doming of the aortic valve is a sensitive sign of stenosis (Fig. 23-1). The valve cusps do not separate in systole, but rather move up and down the outflow area as a fused unit. In diastole, the valve may prolapse into the LV outflow tract due to poor commissural support. Often this is accompanied by aortic regurgitation.

Fig. 23-1. Parasternal long-axis view of stenotic aortic valve. The valve domes in systole. *ao* = aortic root; *lv* = left ventricle.

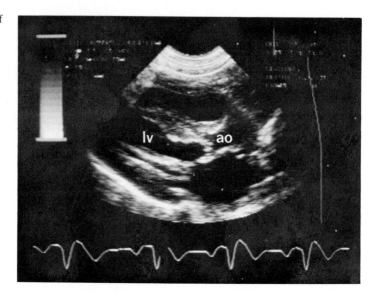

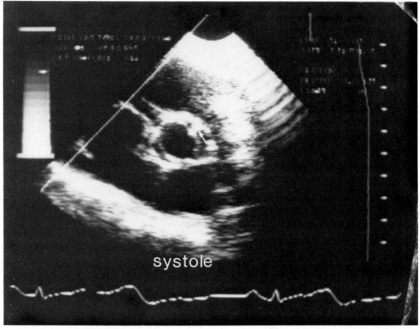

A

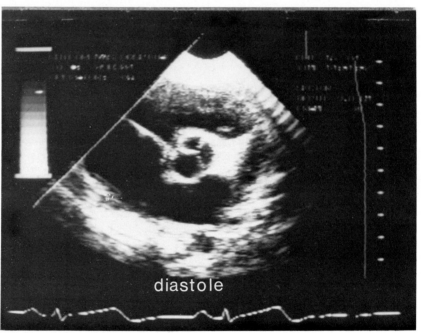

B

Fig. 23-2. Parasternal short-axis view of bicommissural aortic valve in systole (A) and diastole (B). Note that although the abortive raphe (*arrow*) indicates a "Mercedes-Benz sign" in diastole, there are only two functioning commissures seen in systole.

PART III. Obstructive Lesions

The number of commissures is best determined from a parasternal short-axis view of the aortic valve. Cusp motion must be observed in systole to determine the number of commissures accurately. In the tricommissural valve, three hinge points can be seen at the valve annulus, and the cusps separate along cleavage lines directed toward the hinge points. Only two such hinge points can be seen in the bicommissural valve. When open, the cusps circumscribe an oval or ellipse (Fig. 23-2A, B). The raphe can often be seen in the larger cusp, running perpendicular to the plane of cusp separation. In the unicommissural valve, the sole commissure runs in the direction of what in normal patients would be between the left and noncoronary cusps (Fig. 23-3). It usually appears as an eccentric, teardrop-shaped orifice running from the center of the root to the annulus at about 5 o'clock. The diastolic appearance of the valve may be misleading in determining the number of commissures since a raphe and a commissure have a similar appearance in diastole (see Fig. 23-2B). Even a bicommissural valve has three cusps; the problem is really the absence of the commissure.

Fig. 23-3. Parasternal short-axis view of unicommissural valve in a neonate with critical aortic stenosis. Note the teardrop-shaped, eccentric orifice (*arrow*). *ao* = aortic root.

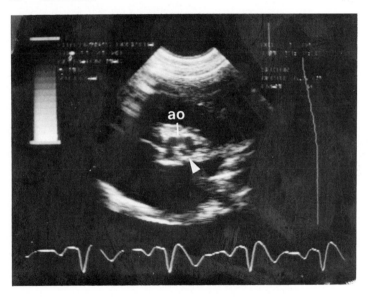

INDIRECT FINDINGS

The degree of LV hypertrophy generally parallels the severity of compensated ventricular pressure overload. LV posterior-wall thickness and transverse dimension, measured in end-systole by M-mode, correlate with LV pressure in patients with valvar aortic stenosis.

Infants with critical aortic stenosis and congestive heart failure may have a dilated, thin-walled LV with poor wall motion as indicated by M-mode or two-dimensional (2-D) studies. In other infants, the LV is a small thick-walled structure. Unusually bright echoes from the endocardial surface and papillary muscles may indicate endocardial fibroelastosis. This phenomenon occurs because the endocardial surface is smooth, due to the absence of the usual fine trabeculations.

Fusiform dilation of the proximal ascending aorta is often present in older children and adults with valvar aortic stenosis (Fig. 23-4). This finding is not related to the severity of obstruction. The ascending aorta may be hypoplastic in infants with critical aortic stenosis or stenosis associated with other intracardiac abnormalities, especially multiple left heart obstructive lesions.

Fig. 23-4. Subxiphoid long-axis view of the left ventricle (*LV*) and ascending aorta (*Asc Ao*) in a patient with valvar aortic stenosis. Note the mild fusiform dilatation of the Asc Ao. *RA* = right atrium; *RVI* = right ventricular inflow.

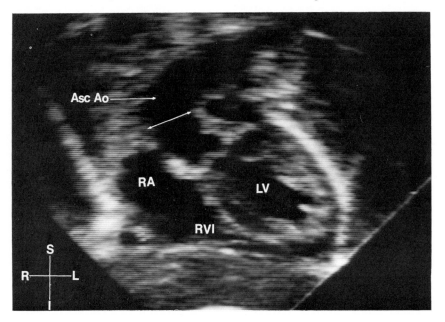

EXAMINATION
TECHNIQUE

Long-axis views of the LV outflow tract (e.g., parasternal, apical, and subxiphoid) demonstrate doming of the aortic valve. The parasternal short-axis view cuts across the valve face, demonstrating the commissures. LV size, wall thickness, and motion may be described from a combination of long- and short-axis views from the parasternal, apical, and subxiphoid positions. M-mode recording of the LV at its equatorial axis (best selected from a 2-D image) provide useful additional information regarding wall thickness and motion.

PROBLEMS

The occasional patient has equivocal clinical findings for bicuspid aortic valve and mild asymmetry noted on 2-D and/or M-mode examination. The distinction between minor asymmetry of the valve and mild pathologic abnormality is vague. The presence of doming of the valves on long axis is an arbitrary, but easily recognized pathologic sign.

All commissures may not be seen simultaneously if the plane of the echo beam is not exactly in the short axis of the aortic valve. Therefore, frame-by-frame review of multiple short-axis sweeps may be required in order to distinguish between a bicuspid and tricuspid aortic valve.

BIBLIOGRAPHY

Bierman, F. Z., Yeh, M. N., Swersky, S., et al. Absence of the aortic valve: Antenatal and postnatal two-dimensional and Doppler echocardiographic features. *J. Am. Coll. Cardiol.* 3:833, 1984.

Brandenburg, R. O., Jr., Tajik, A. J., Edwards, W. D., et al. Accuracy of 2-dimensional echocardiographic diagnosis of congenitally bicuspid aortic valve: Echocardiographic-anatomic correlation in 115 patients. *Am. J. Cardiol.* 51:1469, 1983.

DeMaria, A. N., Bommer, W., Joye, J., et al. Valve and limitations of cross-sectional echocardiography of the aortic valve in the diagnosis and quantification of valvular aortic stenosis. *Circulation* 62:304, 1980.

Radford, D. J., Bloom, K. R., Izukawa, T., et al. Echocardiographic assessment of bicuspid aortic valves: Angiographic and pathological correlates. *Circulation* 53:80, 1976.

CHAPTER 23. Valvar Aortic Stenosis

Coarctation of the Aorta

ANATOMY

The discrete, simple coarctation is usually a short-segment constriction of the aorta, immediately distal to the left subclavian artery, followed by post-stenotic dilation. The outer curve of the aorta is indented at the point of constriction. This curve, with the stenotic dilation of the descending aorta, creates the characteristic "3" sign of coarctation seen on plain chest radiograph. This form of discrete or simple coarctation is often associated with a bicommissural aortic valve.

The long-segment coarctation includes tubular hypoplasia of the transverse aortic arch in addition to a discrete narrowing or shelf at the site of the junction with the ductus arteriosus or diverticulum. The ductus arteriosus may be patent or closed and, if patent, opens into the area of greatest constriction. Long-segment coarctation is almost always associated with intracardiac anomalies: the malalignment type of ventricular septal defect (VSD), subaortic stenosis, single ventricle, double outlet right ventricle (DORV), or other conotruncal abnormalities.

DIAGNOSTIC ECHO FINDINGS

The coarcted segment of aorta must be visualized directly. In both discrete and long-segment coarctation, an indentation is seen along the outer curvature of the aorta. In patients with discrete coarctation, this posterior indentation followed by dilation of the descending aorta creates a "3" sign similar to that seen on plain chest radiograph (Fig. 24-1). The aortic isthmus may be hypoplastic or nearly normal (Fig. 24-2A, B). Doppler examination reveals a high-velocity jet at the site of greatest constriction in patients with discrete obstruction, unless the patient is in low output state. In almost all patients, low-velocity, damped or nonpulsatile flow may be detected in the abdominal descending aorta. A patent ductus arteriosus (PDA) or ductus diverticulum may be seen in young infants (Fig. 24-3).

EXAMINATION TECHNIQUE

The aortic arch must be visualized within the transducer's focal range. For short-focused transducers, the suprasternal notch (SSN) or high parasternal views must be used. Extended focal range transducers usually provide good resolution of the aortic arch from the subxiphoid position in infants, but the region of interest may be obscured by shadowing from the left mainstem bronchus. A view midway between long- and short-axis subxiphoid views will demonstrate the aortic arch. The gain should be varied during the examination. A low-gain setting shows the lumen of the aorta to best advantage.

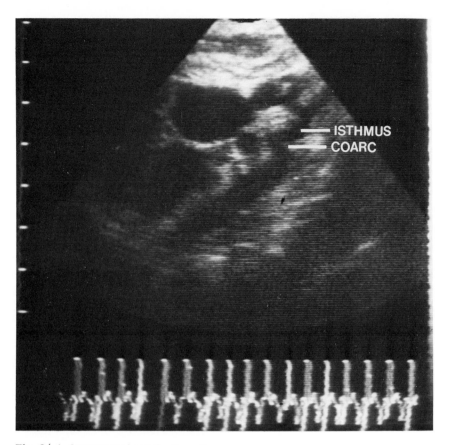

Fig. 24-1. Suprasternal notch view of typical discrete coarctation of the aorta shows indentation of outer curve of the aorta at the site of the coarctation (*COARC*).

CHAPTER 24. Coarctation of the Aorta

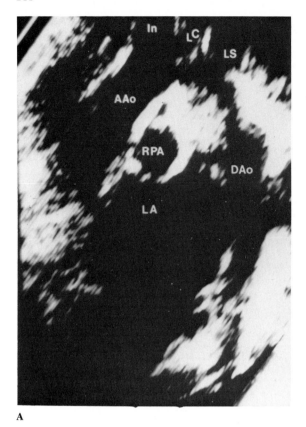
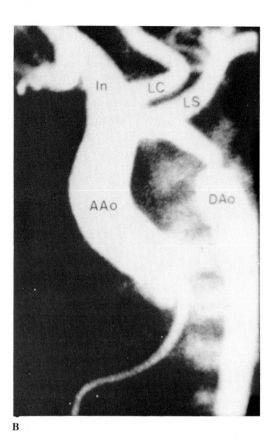

A

B

Fig. 24-2. Suprasternal notch echocardiogram (A) and angiogram (B) (of right ventricle) in a patient with coarctation of the aorta and tubular hypoplasia of the aortic arch. Note that there is a discrete construction as the distal aortic arch joins the descending aorta (*DAo*), and the arch distal to the left subclavian artery (*LS*) is small. *AAo* = ascending aorta; *In* = innominate artery; *LA* = left atrium; *LC* = left carotid artery; *RPA* = right pulmonary artery. (The authors are grateful to Dr. Thomas G. DiSessa for this illustration.)

PROBLEMS

Tortuosity of the aorta at the level of the subclavian artery may cause the lumen to curve out of the beam path, creating a false appearance of coarctation or interruption of the aortic arch. In both situations, the absence of a posterior indentation suggests that coarctation is not present and continued trials of angulation from different transducer positions should reveal the true lumen.

A discrete coarctation of the aorta may not be visualized unless there is good axial and lateral resolution. A PDA lying close to the area of coarctation may appear to overlap the lumen of the aorta, particularly when lateral resolution is poor.

For all these reasons, unless resolution at the level of aortic arch and left subclavian artery is excellent and multiple views are obtained, the likelihood of either false-positive or false-negative diagnosis is significant.

PART III. Obstructive Lesions

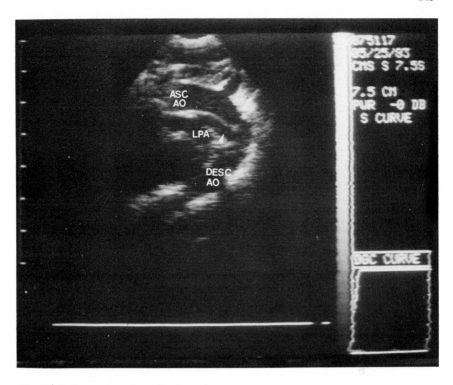

Fig. 24-3. Suprasternal notch view of aortic arch. In this patient with coarctation, a patent ductus arteriosus (*arrow*) overlies the narrowed aortic segment. *ASC AO* = ascending aorta; *DESC AO* = descending aorta; *LPA* = left pulmonary artery.

BIBLIOGRAPHY

Huhta, J. C., Gutgesell, H. P., Latson, L. A., et al. Two-dimensional echocardiographic assessment of the aorta in infants and children with congenital heart disease. *Circulation* 70:417, 1984.

Parr, G. V. S., Waldhausen, J. A., Bharati, S., et al. Coarctation in Taussig-Bing malformation of the heart. Surgical significance. *J. Thorac. Cardiovasc. Surg.* 86:280, 1983.

Riggs, T. W., Berry, T. E., Aziz, K. U., et al. Two-dimensional echocardiographic features of interruption of the aortic arch. *Am. J. Cardiol.* 50:1385, 1982.

Roberts, W. C., Morrow, A. G., and Brownwald, E. Complete interruption of the aortic arch. *Circulation* 26:39, 1962.

Robinson, P. J., Wyse, R. K., Deanfield, J. E., et al. Continuous wave Doppler velocimetry as an adjunct to cross-sectional echocardiography in the diagnosis of critical left heart obstruction in neonates. *Br. Heart J.* 52:552, 1984.

Smallhorn, J. F., et al. Cross-sectional echocardiographic assessment of coarctation in the sick neonate and infant. *Br. Heart J.* 50:349, 1983.

Weyman, A. E., Caldwell, R. L., Hurwitz, R. A., et al. Cross-sectional characterization of aortic obstruction: II. Coarctation of the aorta. *Circulation* 57:498, 1978.

Interrupted Aortic Arch

ANATOMY

The aortic arch may be interrupted distal to the left carotid artery, the left subclavian artery, or innominate artery (in order of decreasing frequency) (Fig. 25-1). The patient is alive by virtue of a patent ductus arteriosus (PDA), which may be widely patent or constricted. Interrupted aortic arch (IAA) is associated with ventricular septal defect (VSD), subaortic obstruction, single ventricle, and conotruncal abnormalities. Interruption of the arch between the carotid arteries is extremely rare and usually associated with severe intracardiac and arterial anomalies. When IAA accompanies truncus arteriosus, the ascending aortic portion of the truncus is small in comparison to the pulmonary artery (PA) component, a reverse of the proportions found in truncus arteriosus without IAA (see Chap. 32).

DIAGNOSTIC ECHO FINDINGS

Complete interruption of the aorta is represented by a gap or discontinuity of the aorta in the area distal to the subclavian artery, left carotid artery, or innominate artery (Fig. 25-2A, B). A PDA connects the main pulmonary artery (MPA) to the descending aorta (Fig. 25-3).

Fig. 25-1. Diagram of interrupted aortic arch with interruption distal to left carotid artery (one of the more common types). The ascending aorta (*Asc. ao.*), smaller than the main pulmonary artery (*PA*), branches into the right innominate and right carotid arteries, producing a V sign. The aortic arch is absent. Instead, a patent ductus arteriosus (*PDA*) arches between the main PA and descending aorta (*Desc. ao.*). *LSA* = left subclavian artery.

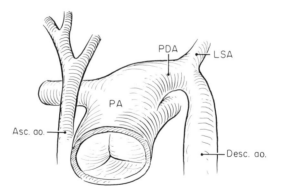

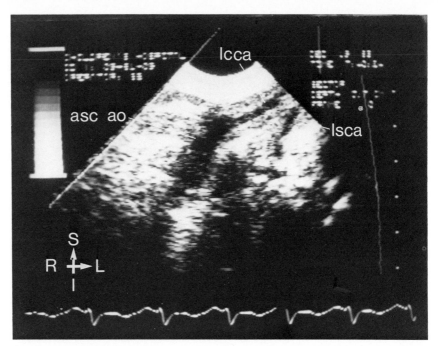

A

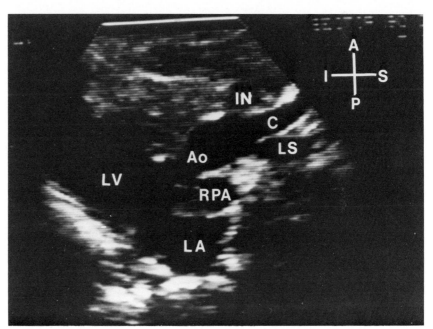

B

Fig. 25-2. (A) Suprasternal notch view of interrupted aortic arch with a break distal to the left carotid artery (*lcca*). Note the smooth left border of the lcca and that there is no vestige of an aortic arch. The left subclavian artery (*lsca*) can be seen separately from the aorta and lcca. (B) High parasternal view of the aorta and brachiocephalic artery with interruption of the aortic arch distal to the left subclavian (*LS*) artery. *Ao* = aorta; *asc ao* = ascending aorta; *IN* = innominate artery; *LA* = left atrium; *LV* = left ventricle; *RPA* = right pulmonary artery.

CHAPTER 25. Interrupted Aortic Arch

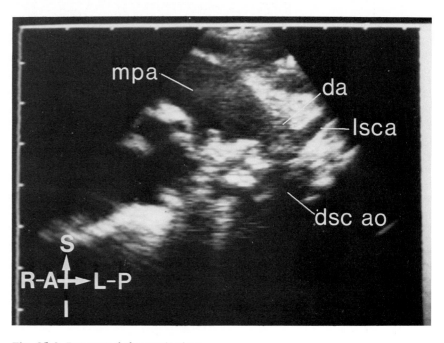

Fig. 25-3. Parasternal short-axis view of the main pulmonary artery (*mpa*) showing the ductus arteriosus (*da*) continuing to the descending aorta (*dsc ao*). The left subclavian artery (*lsca*) can be seen arising from the dsc ao.

EXAMINATION
TECHNIQUE

The suprasternal notch (SSN) view, which usually displays the aortic arch, will show only the ascending aorta and those brachiocephalic vessels arising from it. If the interruption is between the left carotid and left subclavian arteries, the ascending aorta terminates at the left carotid artery. Sweeping across the plane of the ascending aorta shows no segment of transverse arch turning posteriorly to join the descending aorta. The left subclavian artery can usually be seen arising from the descending aorta at its junction with the ductus arteriosus. When the interruption is distal to the left subclavian artery, a portion of the transverse arch is present and courses posteriorly to give rise to the left subclavian artery. However, the distal portion of the transverse arch is absent, and the distal arch and the descending aorta are clearly discontinuous.

PROBLEMS

A PDA may simulate an aortic arch. However, the PAs arise from the proximal segment of this vessel (the MPA) and no brachiocephalic vessels arise from the top of the ductus arteriosus.

PART III. Obstructive Lesions

In atresia of the aortic arch, there is no discontinuity between the two segments of the aorta, but the lumen is obliterated for a variable distance. This may be difficult to differentiate from severe coarctation of the aorta except by Doppler examination. As in coarctation of the aorta, suboptimal lateral and axial resolution and the close proximity of the PDA may cause diagnostic errors.

BIBLIOGRAPHY

Riggs, T. W., Berry, T. E., Aziz, K. U., et al. Two-dimensional echocardiographic features of interruption of the aortic arch. *Am. J. Cardiol.* 50:1385, 1982.

Smallhorn, J. F., Anderson, R. H., and Macartney, F. J. Cross-sectional echocardiographic recognition of interruption of aortic arch between left carotid and subclavian arteries. *Br. Heart J.* 48:229, 1982.

Conotruncal Abnormalities

General Features of Conotruncal Abnormalities

ANATOMY

The major conotruncal abnormalities share certain anatomic features, including abnormal development of the conus or infundibulum (the segment that connects the great arteries and the ventricles). The presence or absence of conus muscle beneath a semilunar valve determines in part the position of a great artery and its alignment with the ventricles. There are four major conotruncal abnormalities, with a myriad of anatomic variations: tetralogy of Fallot, truncus arteriosus, transposition of the great arteries (TGA), and double outlet right ventricle (DORV). Intermediate forms of these anomalies engender much debate among practitioners of the different diagnostic modalities.

The presence and size of conus muscle beneath a semilunar valve largely determines its relative anteroposterior (A-P) and superoinferior spatial relations. When no conus muscle is present, a semilunar valve is posterior and inferior, sitting directly above the atrioventricular (A-V) valves. The presence of conus muscle between the semilunar root and the A-V valve ring displaces the semilunar root anteriorly and superiorly. The degree of displacement is proportional to the amount of conus muscle present beneath the valve. If the displacement is slight, the semilunar root retains its alignment with the posterior ventricle; if the conus muscle is fully expanded, the semilunar root is usually aligned with the more anterior ventricle. The infundibular, or outflow, septum normally joins the lower (trabecular) muscular septum at a slight angle. Abnormal location of the infundibular septum is usually associated with the following: (1) a malalignment type of ventricular septal defect (VSD), (2) the overriding of a semilunar root, (3) encroachment on either the pulmonary or aortic outflow tract, depending on the position of the great arteries and direction of displacement of the infundibular septum, and (4) disproportion between the great arteries with hypoplasia of the great artery arising from the narrowed outflow tract and dilatation of the overriding great artery. As an example, tetralogy of Fallot is characterized by anterior and leftward shift of the infundibular septum, with narrowing of the subpulmonary area, a malalignment VSD, and a large, overriding aorta.

In the normal or d-ventricular loop, the morphologic right ventricle (RV) is to the right of the morphologic left ventricle (LV), and the aortic annulus is to the right of the pulmonary annulus (with occasional exceptions). In the following chapters, we will refer to this arrangement as d-loop, and this will be implied unless specified otherwise. The ventricular and great artery right-left relations are reversed in the typical patient with ventricular inversion or l-loop. Although many positional variations of the ventricles and great arteries are possible, we will refer to the most common alignments for the sake of clarity.

The aims of the echocardiographer are to define (1) the position of the great arteries relative to the interventricular septum (IVS) and VSD, if present, (2) the position of the infundibular septum relative to the lower trabecular IVS, (3) the origin of the major branches of the great arteries, and (4) the presence of associated lesions.

The positions of the ventricles, conus arteriosus, and great arteries are so variable that one cannot outline a prescribed sequence of transducer positions for their display. However, there is an orderly process whereby the pertinent anatomic relationships are defined. First, determine the relative positions of the ventricles by A-V valve morphology and attachments, ventricular morphology, and papillary muscle position (see Chap. 30). Note the position of the infundibular chamber, which almost always rises over the RV, but may straddle the IVS or relate to the LV in rare circumstances.

Next, find a transducer position that displays both great arteries simultaneously and the long axis of the anterior great artery. Such a view may be a subxiphoid long-axis view of the right ventricular outflow tract (S4) or a high parasternal transverse view. This view will automatically demonstrate the infundibular septum, which divides the subpulmonary and subaortic regions. Note the position of the infundibular septum relative to the midmuscular IVS by sweeping from one structure to the other if necessary.

Define the ventricular origin of each great artery. A great artery is considered to arise from a ventricle if more than 50 percent of the semilunar annulus rises above it. The midmuscular septum is a reference point from which the position of an overriding great artery is judged. Under the most favorable circumstances, a transducer position can be selected that simultaneously displays the long axes of the great artery and the midmuscular septum. The same information can be obtained by sweeping in serial cross sections from the semilunar root to the septum below, but this technique is subject to error in approximation since both structures are not viewed simultaneously.

Determine VSD location by multiple-plane scanning (see Chap. 6). The defect usually lies beneath the more posterior of the two great arteries, but may be found in the muscular or A-V (canal) septum instead.

Assess the presence of conus muscle under each semilunar root directly by observation and indirectly by inference from the position of the semilunar valve. Conus muscle can be observed from a transducer position that displays the posterior border of the semilunar root and the nearest A-V valve. For example, the parasternal long-axis and the apical 2-chamber views demonstrate conus muscle, if present, between the posterior semilunar root and proximal attachment of the anterior mitral leaflet. Indirectly, one may usually assume that an anterior and superior position of a semilunar root suggests the presence of conus muscle beneath it, although there are exceptions.

The following chapters will describe the standard appearances of the most common forms of conotruncal abnormalities. In many complex malpositions, positions of the great arteries are ambiguous, particularly when

CHAPTER 26. General Features of Conotruncal Abnormalities

one of the great vessels is atretic. In these situations, a clear description of the position of the great arteries relative to the IVS and the VSD, if present, is more helpful in preoperative assessment than a strict categorizaton.

BIBLIOGRAPHY

Gutgesell, H. P., Huhta, J. C., Cohen, M. H., et al. Two-dimensional echocardiographic assessment of pulmonary artery and aortic arch anatomy in cyanotic infants. *J. Am. Coll. Cardiol.* 4:1242, 1984.

Hagler, D. J., Tajik, A. J., Seward, J. B., et al. Wide-angle two-dimensional echocardiographic profiles of conotruncal abnormalities. *Mayo Clin. Proc.* 55:73, 1980.

Maron, B. J., Henry, W. L., Griffith, J. M., et al. Identification of congenital malformations of the great arteries in infants by real-time two-dimensional echocardiography. *Circulation* 52:671, 1975.

Sanders, S. P., Bierman, F. Z., and Williams, R. G. Conotruncal malformations: Diagnosis in infancy using subxiphoid two-dimensional echocardiography. *Am. J. Cardiol.* 50:1361, 1982.

Tetralogy of Fallot

ANATOMY

Tetralogy of Fallot is characterized by anterior, superior, and leftward displacement of the infundibular septum (i.e., outflow septum, parietal band, crista supraventricularis) with respect to the lower muscular septum (Fig. 27-1A, B). Since the infundibular septum forms the back wall of the right ventricular (RV) outflow tract, this channel is narrowed unless there is expansion of the anterior free wall. Usually the opposite is true: the infundibular free wall is somewhat hypoplastic, further contributing to the subpulmonary obstruction. This subpulmonary obstruction is associated with hypoplasia of the pulmonary annulus as well as the main (MPA) and branch pulmonary arteries (PAs). Displacement of the infundibular septum from the "y" of septal band creates a malalignment type of ventricular septal defect (VSD), which is typically large (Fig. 27-2A, B). Through it, the aorta overrides the interventricular septum (IVS). The aorta is usually dilated, its anterior border lying over the RV, while its posterior border maintains its normal position in fibrous continuity with the mitral annulus. In some cases, the intervalvular fibrosa (fibrous tissue between the mitral and aortic annuli) may be attenuated, resulting in minor anterior displacement of the posterior border of the aortic root, but this displacement is to a milder degree than that encountered in double outlet right ventricle (DORV). Also, in contrast with DORV, there is little or no conus muscle interposed between the two fibrous annuli in tetralogy of Fallot.

Fig. 27-1. (A) Drawing of long axis of right ventricle (*RV*) as seen from the left in a normal heart. This cut is similar to the subxiphoid short-axis (S4) view. The infundibular septum (*stippled*) forms a smooth, unbroken curve with the trabecular septum (*striped*). (B) Drawing of similar view of RV in tetralogy of Fallot. The infundibular septum is tilted upward and anteriorly, losing its connection with the lower trabecular septum and narrowing the right ventricular outflow tract. Note the horizontal positions of the right ventricular outflow tract and main pulmonary artery (*MPA*), compared with normal. *LV* = left ventricle; *MV* = mitral valve.

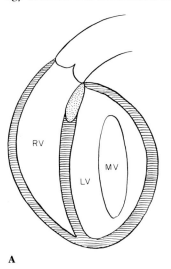

A

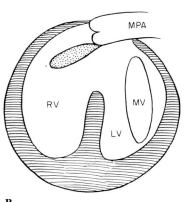

B

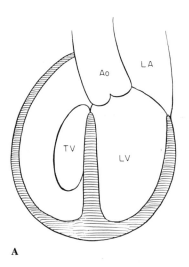
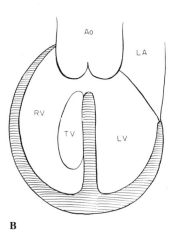

A   B

Fig. 27-2. (A) Drawing of the left ventricular outflow tract in a normal patient as seen from subxiphoid short-axis (S3) view. The ascending aorta curves posteriorly to rise from the left ventricle (*LV*). The anterior border of the aortic root (*Ao*) is continuous with the interventricular septum. (B) Similar drawing in tetralogy of Fallot. The di-lated aortic root straddles the interventricular septum. The anterior border of the aortic root is no longer continuous with the interventricular septum, but the posterior border is continuous with the mitral annulus. *LA* = left atrium; *RV* = right ventricle; *TV* = tricuspid valve.

Occasionally, a variation of tetralogy of Fallot is encountered in which the infundibular septum is hypoplastic as well as displaced. In such cases, the subaortic (malalignment) VSD extends under the pulmonary valve as well and the pulmonary annulus is lower than is usually found in tetralogy of Fallot. This finding has relevance to surgical repair.

A very rare diagnosis, often confused with tetralogy of Fallot and having important implications for surgical repair, is double outlet left ventricle (DOLV) of the tetralogy-of-Fallot type. In this type of DOLV, the pulmonary valve is more inferior and posterior than usual, arising from the LV. The overriding aortic root and subpulmonary obstruction in this type of DOLV mimic the more commonplace tetralogy of Fallot.

DIAGNOSTIC ECHO FINDINGS

The RV outflow tract is narrowed by anterior displacement of its posterior wall, the infundibular septum. This narrowing gives the outflow tract and MPA a more horizontal orientation than usual (Fig. 27-3A, B).

The MPA and branches are mildly to severely hypoplastic. Some degree of pulmonary arterial hypoplasia is noted even when there is only mild RV outflow obstruction (Fig. 27-4A, B).

The usual malalignment VSD lies superior to the tricuspid valve (tricuspid attachment to the papillary muscle of the conus) and immediately below the aortic valve cusps, but the defect may extend medially into the inflow septum or laterally into the subpulmonic area.

PART IV. Conotruncal Abnormalities

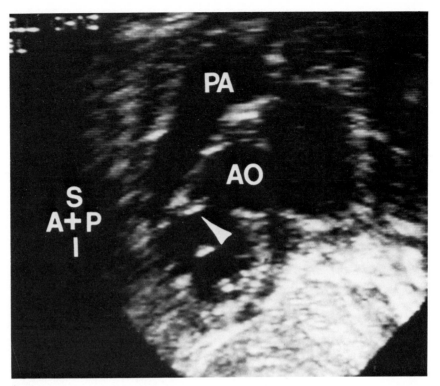

A

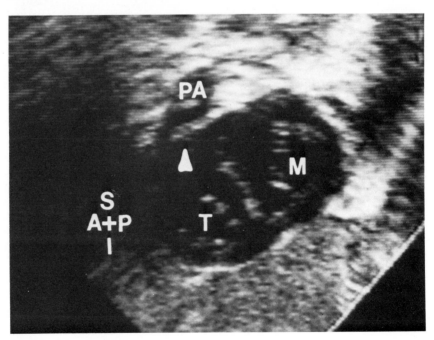

B

Fig. 27-3. View similar to Figure 27-1B in patients with mild (A) and severe (B) tetralogy of Fallot. The right ventricular outflow tract is narrowed by the displaced infundibular septum (*arrows*). This gives the right ventricular outflow tract a more horizontal position than normal. *AO* = aortic root; *M* = mitral valve; *PA* = pulmonary artery; *T* = tricuspid valve.

CHAPTER 27. Tetralogy of Fallot

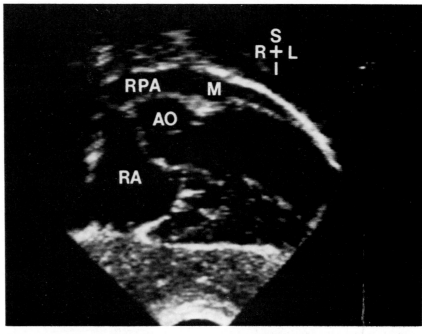

A

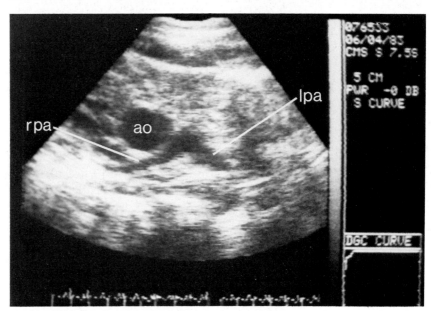

B

Fig. 27-4. (A) Subxiphoid long-axis view (superior angulation from a 4-chamber view) of the pulmonary arteries in a patient with mild tetralogy of Fallot. The distal main (*M*) and branch right pulmonary arteries (*RPA*) are visualized. (B) High parasternal short-axis view of the small main and branch pulmonary arteries in tetralogy of Fallot with pulmonary atresia. *AO, ao* = aortic root; *lpa* = left pulmonary artery; *RA* = right atrium; *rpa* = right pulmonary artery.

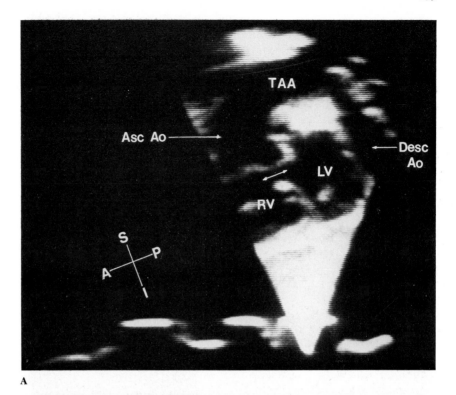

A

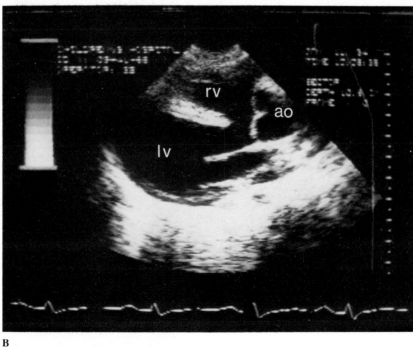

B

Fig. 27-5. Subxiphoid short-axis (S3) (A) and parasternal long-axis (B) views of an overriding aorta in tetralogy of Fallot. Note ventricular septal defect (*double-headed arrow*). *ao* = aortic root; *Asc Ao* = ascending aorta; *Desc Ao* = descending aorta; *LV*, *lv* = left ventricle; *RV*, *rv* = right ventricle; *TAA* = transverse aortic arch.

CHAPTER 27. Tetralogy of Fallot

The anterior border of the aortic root lies above the RV, while its posterior border is in its usual position above the anterior mitral leaflet (Fig. 27-5A, B). The aortic root is large, inversely proportional to the size of the pulmonary root. Occasionally, the aortic cusps are thickened or abnormal in number, which may be associated with signs of aortic regurgitation.

Hypertrophy of the RV free wall is present.

VARIATIONS

1. A right aortic arch is frequently associated (25% of cases) with tetralogy of Fallot (Fig. 27-6).
2. The RV infundibulum may be hypoplastic, allowing the upper margin of the VSD to extend nearly or completely to the pulmonary annulus.
3. There may be minor degrees of anterior displacement of the posterior aortic root without interposed subaortic conus.
4. An atrial septal defect (ASD) may be present.
5. Anomalous RV muscle bundles may be associated with tetralogy of Fallot, producing outflow obstruction at two levels.
6. Rarely, tetralogy of Fallot is associated with complete A-V canal, aortic or subaortic stenosis, or aortic regurgitation.

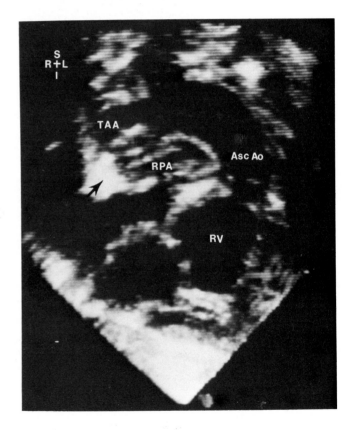

Fig. 27-6. Subxiphoid long-axis view of right aortic arch angulated superiorly to show coronal section of right ventricle (*RV*) in a patient with tetralogy of Fallot. A dilated aorta (with biventricular origin) arises partially from the RV and curves to the right to pass over the right mainstem bronchus (*arrow*). The right pulmonary artery (*RPA*) is visualized beneath the curve of the aortic arch. Compare this illustration with Figure 27-5A, which demonstrates a typical left aortic arch. *Asc Ao* = ascending aorta; *TAA* = transverse aortic arch.

EXAMINATION
TECHNIQUES

The examination is first focused on display of the malaligned infundibular septum and RV outflow tract. Anterior displacement of the infundibular septum is best displayed by views that display the long axis of RV outflow: the subxiphoid short-axis (S4) position and the high transverse parasternal view. Right-left narrowing of the RV outflow tract may be demonstrated on a coronal view of the RV from the subxiphoid (L4) view, which shows the leftward displacement of the infundibular septum.

Overriding of the aorta relative to the ventricular septum is displayed from transducer positions with anteroposterior (A-P) coordinates: the parasternal long-axis, apical 2-chamber, and subxiphoid (S3) views.

The origin of the MPA from the RV is demonstrated from views that display the long axis of RV outflow: subxiphoid short-axis (S4) and high transverse parasternal views. The continuity of the MPA and right and left branches is demonstrated by views that display right-left coordinates: subxiphoid long-axis views as well as high transverse parasternal and suprasternal views. The long axis of the right pulmonary artery (RPA) is displayed from these views. Only the proximal left pulmonary artery (LPA) is seen from these views because this structure dives posteriorly. Since LPA has a posterior course, it is better displayed from subxiphoid (S4) and high transverse parasternal views, which have A-P coordinates.

PROBLEMS

When the RV outflow tract is extremely narrowed, it is sometimes difficult to assess patency. Doppler study may be employed to determine the presence or absence of antegrade flow in the MPA.

Although the MPA and RPA are easily displayed, it is sometimes difficult to recognize obstruction at the junction between the MPA and LPA.

Anomalous origin of the left anterior descending coronary artery from the right coronary artery is an occasional finding in patients with tetralogy of Fallot that usually precludes placement of a patch across the pulmonary annulus. Identification of this problem requires extensive experience in recognizing the coronary branching pattern.

Some patients have a malalignment VSD without significant RV outflow obstruction. Although these patients may present with congestive heart failure, some develop typical anatomic and physiologic features of tetralogy of Fallot with time. In these patients, terminology may be confusing.

As mentioned previously, one type of DOLV (a very rare lesion) has the superficial appearance of tetralogy of Fallot. This lesion is recognized by the relatively inferior and posterior position of the pulmonary annulus, best seen by scanning from subxiphoid long-axis views of the RV outflow tract.

CHAPTER 27. Tetralogy of Fallot

BIBLIOGRAPHY

Bharati, S., Lev, M., Stewart, R., et al. The morphologic spectrum of double outlet left ventricle and its surgical significance. *Circulation* 58:558, 1978.

Celano, V., Pieroni, D. R., Gingell, R. L., et al. Two-dimensional recognition of the right aortic arch. *Am. J. Cardiol.* 51:1507, 1983.

Huhta, J. C., Piehler, J. M., Tajik, A. J., et al. Two-dimensional echocardiographic detection and measurement of the right pulmonary artery in pulmonary atresia–ventricular septal defect: Angiographic and surgical correlation. *Am. J. Cardiol.* 49:1235, 1982.

Lappen, R. S., Riggs, T. W., Lapen, G. D., et al. Two-dimensional echocardiographic measurement of right pulmonary artery diameter in infants and children. *J. Am. Coll. Cardiol.* 2:121, 1983.

Lewis, B. S., Amitae, N., Simche, A., et al. Echocardiographic diagnosis of pulmonary atresia with interventricular septum. *Am. Heart J.* 97:92, 1979.

Morris, D. C., Felner, J. M., Schlant, R. C., et al. Echocardiographic diagnosis of tetralogy of Fallot. *Am. J. Cardiol.* 36:908, 1975.

Tinker, P. D., Nanda, N. C., Harris, J. P., et al. Two dimensional echocardiographic identification of pulmonary artery branch block stenosis. *Am. J. Cardiol.* 50:814, 1982.

CHAPTER 28

Absent Pulmonary Valve Syndrome (with Tetralogy of Fallot)

ANATOMY

Despite the name *absent pulmonary valve syndrome*, vestigial pulmonary valve cusps are present in this disorder. The pulmonary annulus may be hypoplastic or dilated. The lesion is rarely isolated, being more commonly associated with a variety of conotruncal abnormalities, especially tetralogy of Fallot. The main pulmonary artery (MPA) and branch pulmonary arteries (PAs) are massively dilated. Significant pulmonary regurgitation also produces right ventricular (RV) dilation.

DIAGNOSTIC ECHO FINDINGS

Absent pulmonary valve syndrome is recognized by massive dilation of the MPA and branch PAs (Fig. 28-1A, B). Remnants of pulmonary cusps may be visible. Typical findings of tetralogy of Fallot are also present (see Chap. 27), but narrowing of the RV outflow tract is usually mild.

Doppler echocardiography demonstrates diastolic retrograde flow in the PAs and RV.

EXAMINATION TECHNIQUE

The pulmonary valve and annulus are displayed from parasternal and subxiphoid short-axis (S4) views of the RV outflow tract. The MPA and left pulmonary artery (LPA) are also displayed from these views. The length of the right pulmonary artery (RPA) is seen from subxiphoid long-axis, suprasternal notch (SSN), and high transverse parasternal views.

PROBLEMS

Severe pulmonary hyperinflation, caused by airway compression from dilated PAs, may severely limit the acoustic window. In many cases, the heart can only be imaged from the subxiphoid position.

Visualization of pulmonary cusp remnants may lead to the erroneous belief that absent pulmonary valve syndrome can be excluded.

BIBLIOGRAPHY

Cheatham, J. B., Latson, L. A., Gutgesell, H. P., et al. Echocardiographic pulsed Doppler features of absent pulmonary valve syndrome in the neonate. *Am. J. Cardiol.* 49:1773, 1982.

DiSegni, E., Emzig, S., Bass, J. L., et al. Congenital absence of the pulmonary valve associated with tetralogy of Fallot: Diagnosis by two-dimensional echocardiography. *Am. J. Cardiol.* 51:1978, 1983.

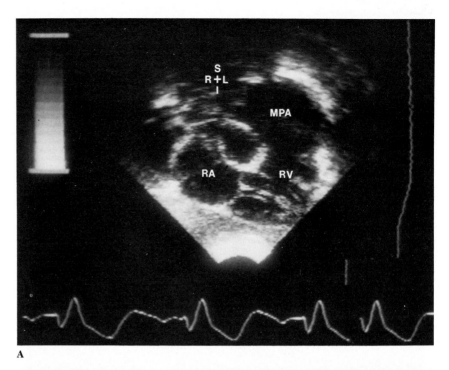

A

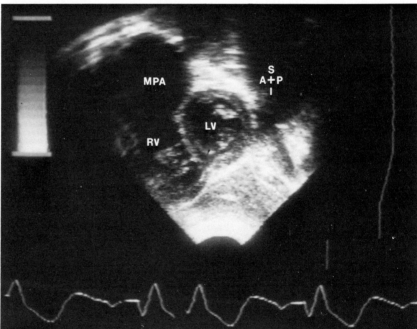

B

Fig. 28-1. (A) Subxiphoid long-axis view with extreme superior angulation shows dilated main (*MPA*) and right pulmonary arteries in a patient with absent pulmonary valve syndrome, associated with tetralogy of Fallot. This massive dilatation of the pulmonary arteries is characteristic of this lesion. (B) Companion subxiphoid short-axis view (S4) demonstrates size of right ventricle (*RV*) and MPA relative to left ventricle (*LV*). *RA* = right atrium.

PART IV. Conotruncal Abnormalities

Simple or D-Transposition of the Great Arteries

ANATOMY

In D-transposition of the great arteries (D-TGA), the anteroposterior (A-P) position of the great arteries is reversed due to the presence of subaortic conus muscle and the absence of subpulmonic conus muscle. As a result, the anterior aorta arises from the right ventricle (RV) and the posterior pulmonary artery (PA) arises from the left ventricle (LV) (Fig. 29-1A). The aortic valve is also superior to the pulmonary valve, a reversal of the normal situation. Although the aortic valve is usually to the right of the PA, it may lie directly anterior or slightly to the left (Fig. 29-1B to D).

Fig. 29-1. (A) Drawing shows ventriculoarterial alignment in simple D-transposition of the great arteries. The great vessels are parallel as the anterior aorta (*Ao*) rises from the right ventricle (*RV*) and the posterior pulmonary artery (*PA*) from the left ventricle (*LV*).

(B, C, D) Drawings depict the variable great artery positions occurring in D-transposition of the great arteries. Most commonly, the aorta is to the right of the PA (B), but it may lie directly anterior to (C) or slightly to the left of (D) the PA. *LA* = left atrium.

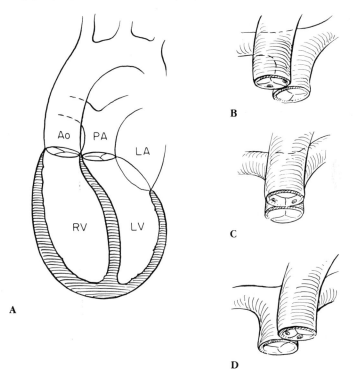

D-TGA may be associated with an intact interventricular septum (IVS) or an interventricular septal defect. A malalignment type of septal defect may be present if the infundibular septum is shifted either anteriorly or posteriorly. A subaortic obstruction may be created by anterior shift of the infundibular septum. This finding may be associated with coarctation of the aorta or interrupted aortic arch. If the infundibular septum is shifted posteriorly, it may narrow the subpulmonary area. Defects may also be found in the membranous atrioventricular (A-V) and trabecular muscular septa.

D-TGA with intact ventricular septum is often associated with mild to moderate dynamic subpulmonary obstruction, thought to be caused by deviation of the IVS toward the LV cavity and potentiated by the small end-systolic cavity size of an LV facing a low PA pressure. This phenomenon becomes more apparent as pulmonary pressure falls in the first days of life and LV pressure falls below that of the RV. Discrete fibrous or fibromuscular subpulmonary obstruction may be present, caused by a subpulmonary membrane, an abnormally placed papillary muscle, or anomalous chordal attachments between the anterior mitral leaflet and IVS.

DIAGNOSTIC ECHO FINDINGS

The aorta, identified by its branching pattern, arises from the morphologic RV. The PA, also identified by its branching pattern, arises from the LV. The morphology of the two ventricles, their connections with the proximal arterial roots, and the branching patterns of the vessels should be directly visualized (Fig. 29-2A, B). If diagnosis relies on indirect inferences from the position of the great arteries, there is a greater likelihood of error because of the wide spectrum of ventriculoarterial relations.

The aortic valve is anterior, superior, and to the right of the pulmonary valve in D-TGA, except in a small number of patients in whom the aorta is directly anterior to or slightly to the left of the PA. The unusual leftward position of the aortic valve should cause no diagnostic confusion if the alignment between ventricles and arteries is directly visualized.

The systolic shape of the IVS is usually straight in the early neonatal period, but within the next few days or weeks, begins to curve into the LV as PA and LV pressures drop below systemic values (Fig. 29-3A, B).

Dynamic subpulmonary stenosis is suggested by bulging of the IVS into the LV outflow tract, accompanied by systolic anterior motion of the mitral valve and fluttering/midsystolic closure of the pulmonary cusps. In fixed subpulmonary stenosis, there may be a subpulmonary membrane, anomalous mitral attachments, or a posteriorly deviated infundibular septum obstructing the subpulmonary area (see Chap. 21).

EXAMINATION TECHNIQUE

The aorta ascends superiorly from the RV and arches posteriorly toward the descending aorta. Consequently, the origin of the aortic root and entire aortic arch may be displayed from a subxiphoid short-axis (S3) view, as seen in

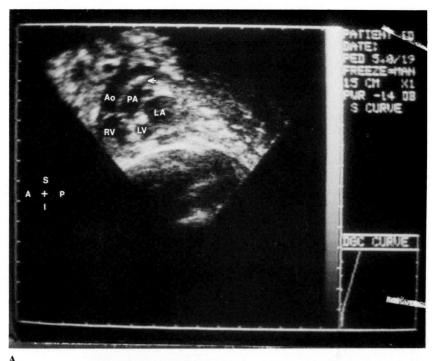

A

Fig. 29-2. (A) Subxiphoid short-axis view in a patient with D-transposition of the great arteries. The ascending portions of the great arteries are parallel, with the aorta (*Ao*) more anterior, arising from the right ventricle (*RV*), and the pulmonary artery (*PA*) more posterior, arising from the left ventricle (*LV*). A patent ductus arteriosus (*arrow*) runs between the main PA and Ao. A ductus is easily visualized in D-transposition of the great arteries because the great arteries are parallel and can be displayed simultaneously. (B) Subxiphoid long-axis (L3) view in a patient with D-transposition of the great arteries. The alignment of the bifurcating main pulmonary artery (*pa*) with the left ventricle (*lv*) is clearly seen in this view, which displays right-left coordinates. *LA* = left atrium; *ra* = right atrium; *RV* = right ventricle.

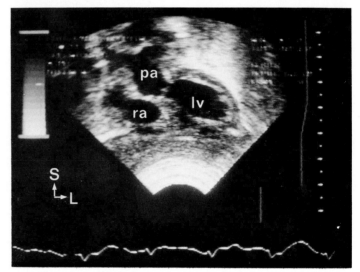

B

CHAPTER 29. Simple or D-Transposition of the Great Arteries

Fig. 29-3. (A) Subxiphoid short-axis view of left ventricle (*LV*). The interventricular septum is straight in a newborn with D-transposition of the great arteries and systemic pulmonary artery pressure. (B) Subxiphoid short-axis view in an older infant with D-transposition of the great arteries and normal pulmonary artery pressure. The interventricular septum now curves into the LV in systole as right ventricular pressure exceeds that of the LV. *RV* = right ventricle.

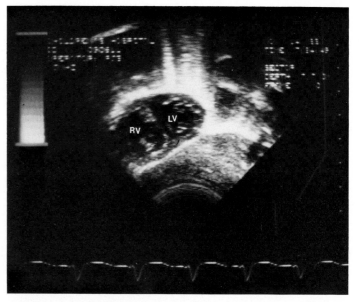

A

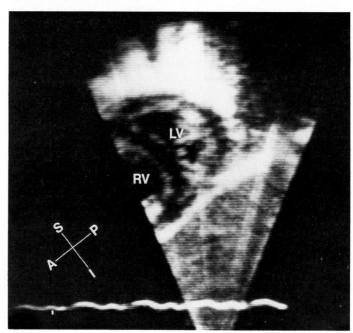

B

Figure 29-2A. The origin of the main pulmonary artery (MPA) from the LV and its bifurcation may be displayed from a subxiphoid long-axis (L3) or an apical 4-chamber view with superior angulation. The subpulmonary area may be displayed from the subxiphoid long-axis (L3) or parasternal long-axis views, but should be examined from all available views in order to recognize a thin subpulmonary membrane or irregular projection from the anterior or medial border of the LV outflow tract. The ventricular septum should be scanned for a defect, as described in Chapter 6.

PROBLEMS

Good lateral resolution at the level of the great arteries is required in order to identify their branching patterns correctly from the subxiphoid approach.

The wide anatomic variations of ventriculoarterial attachments require direct visualization of the origin of the great arteries, best achieved by transducer angulation from the subxiphoid views since the other views do not provide such a flexible acoustic window. The transducer may be rotated, angulated, or moved to the right or left subcostal regions to align the transducer beam with the long axes of the great artery and the ventricle of origin.

Both great arteries must be visualized in order to identify the conotruncal abnormalities correctly. Atresia of a great artery cannot be assumed if only one semilunar root is visualized.

Exclusion of fixed subpulmonary stenosis coexistent with dynamic obstruction is difficult because the LV outflow tract is usually narrowed by the leftward bulging of the IVS.

BIBLIOGRAPHY

Barino, B., de Simone, G., Pasquini, L., et al. Complete transposition of the great arteries: Visualization of left and right outflow obstruction by oblique subcostal two-dimensional echocardiography. *Am. J. Cardiol.* 55:1146, 1985.

Bierman, F. Z., and Williams, R. G. Prospective diagnosis of D-transposition of the great arteries in neonates by subxiphoid, two-dimensional echocardiography. *Circulation* 60:1496, 1979.

Chiu, I., Anderson, R. H., Macartney, F. J., et al. Morphologic features of an intact ventricular septum susceptible to subpulmonary obstruction in complete transposition. *Am. J. Cardiol.* 53:1633, 1984.

Daskapoulas, D. A., Edwards, W. D., Driscoll, D. J., et al. Correlation of two-dimensional echocardiographic and autopsy findings in complete transposition of the great arteries. *J. Am. Coll. Cardiol.* 2:1151, 1983.

Deal, B. J., Chin, A. J., Sanders, S. P., et al. Subxiphoid two-dimensional echocardiographic identification of tricuspid valve abnormalities in transposition of the great arteries. *Am. J. Cardiol.* 55:1146, 1985.

Houston, A. B., Gregory, N. L., and Coleman, E. N. Echocardiographic identification of aorta and main pulmonary artery in complete transposition. *Br. Heart J.* 40:377, 1978.

Huta, J. C., Edwards, W. D., Danielson, G. K., et al. Complete transposition of the great arteries with ventricular septal defect. *J. Thorac. Cardiovasc. Surg.* 83:569, 1982.

King, M. E., Braun, H., Goldblatt, A., et al. Interventricular septal configuration as a predictor of right ventricular systolic hypertension in children: A cross-sectional echocardiographic study. *Circulation* 68:68, 1983.

Moene, R. J., and Oppenheimer-Dekker, A. Congenital mitral valve anomalies in transposition of the great arteries. *Am. J. Cardiol.* 49:1973, 1982.

CHAPTER 29. Simple or D-Transposition of the Great Arteries

Corrected or L-Transposition of the Great Arteries

ANATOMY

Corrected transposition of the great arteries (C-TGA) is also known as L-transposition of the great arteries (L-TGA) or ventricular inversion with atrioventricular (A-V) and ventriculoarterial discordance. In its usual form, atrial situs is normal. Mirror-image looping (to the left) of the primitive heart tube during embryonic development brings the anatomic left ventricle (LV) to the right side, where it receives systemic venous blood from the right atrium (RA) and delivers it to the pulmonary artery (PA) (Fig. 30-1A, B). The anatomic right ventricle (RV), positioned on the left side, receives pulmonary venous (PV) blood from the left atrium (LA). The aorta arises from the anatomic RV via an infundibular chamber. Thus, in the simple form of this anomaly, the circulation of blood is normal, even though the ventricular chambers are reversed.

Unless associated defects cause specific chamber enlargement, the two ventricles lie side by side. Thus, the interventricular septum (IVS) lies in a more nearly sagittal plane than usual.

C-TGA also implies reversal of the position of the great arteries. The PA is rightward, posterior, and inferior, in fibrous continuity with the A-V annulus. The aorta is leftward and arises anteriorly and superiorly from an RV infundibulum. The presence of conus muscle beneath the aortic valve creates discontinuity between aortic annulus and the A-V annulus.

ASSOCIATED LESIONS

Ventricular septal defect (VSD) is a commonly associated anomaly. Often, it is accompanied by valvar or subvalvar pulmonary stenosis. Subvalvar stenosis may be tunnellike or created by accessory tissue associated with the A-V valves. In some cases, this accessory tissue forms a spinnakerlike sail in the subpulmonary area.

Ebstein's anomaly of the left-sided tricuspid valve may occur with C-TGA and is often associated with significant regurgitation into the LA.

C-TGA may be a component of even more complex disease, including abnormalities of visceral and atrial situs, A-V valve atresia, and conotruncal anomalies.

DIAGNOSTIC ECHO FINDINGS

The ventricular loop can be defined by (1) determining the identity and relative positions of the two ventricles and (2) using the "hand rule" to characterize the anatomic RV.

Fig. 30-1. (A) Drawing depicts anatomy of corrected or L-transposition of the great arteries. The right atrium (*RA*) leads to the morphologic left ventricle (*LV*) via the mitral valve (*MV*). The deep septal medial mitral leaflet forms the lateral border of the left ventricular outflow tract. There is mitral-pulmonary continuity. The pulmonary artery (*PA*) rises from the LV in a posterior-rightward and inferior position. The morphologic right ventricle (*RV*) receives left atrial (not seen) blood via the tricuspid valve (*TV*), which is attached along the width of the septal leaflet to the interventricular septum. The aorta (*Ao*) rises from the RV infundibulum in an anterior-leftward and superior position, relative to the PA. (B) A similar subxiphoid long-axis view in patient with corrected transposition of the great arteries. *mv* = mitral valve.

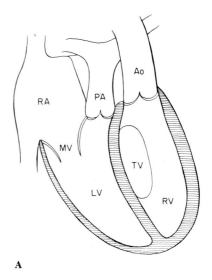

A

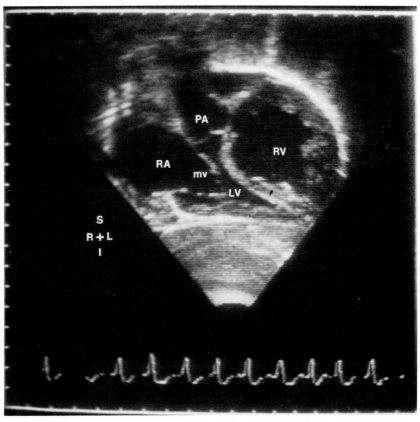

B

CHAPTER 30. Corrected or L-Transposition of the Great Arteries

Ventricular Identity   The identity of each ventricle is defined by using a combination of characteristics of the inflow and outflow tracts and papillary and trabecular muscles, morphology, ventricular shape, and great artery position.

Inflow

1. 4-chamber views of the crux of the heart demonstrate a more apical attachment of the tricuspid annulus to the IVS than the mitral annulus. This attachment is more pronounced when there is Ebstein's anomaly of the tricuspid valve.

   EXCEPTION

   This finding is not present when there is a complete A-V septal defect.

2. The tricuspid valve has three or more leaflets; the septal leaflet is short. The orifice of the tricuspid valve is more round than the mitral valve on short-axis views. The normal mitral valve has two leaflets: a deep septal leaflet and a broad posterior or free-wall leaflet. The orifice has a fishmouth shape.

   EXCEPTIONS

   In the presence of an isolated A-V (inflow) septal defect, the septal tricuspid leaflet may be deep with a pendulous motion.

   A "cleft" mitral valve has three leaflets instead of two, and the orifice is triangular rather than fishmouth-shaped.

3. The septal leaflet of the mitral valve is separated from the IVS by an outflow tract (Fig. 30-2), while the tricuspid valve is not. The entire width of the tricuspid septal leaflet is attached to the IVS.

4. Normally, only the tricuspid valve is attached to the papillary muscle (Lanchesi) of the conus or infundibular septum.

   EXCEPTIONS

   1. A mitral valve that overrides a malalignment VSD may attach to the infundibular septum.

   2. In A-V canal cushion defects, the midportions of the cleft anterior mitral leaflets are attached to the IVS.

Outflow

The RV outflow tract is formed by an infundibular chamber. Hence, the semilunar (aortic, in this case) valve is separated from the A-V (tricuspid) valve (Fig. 30-3). In other words, the A-V valve does not form a lateral border of the immediate subarterial outflow tract of the RV. In contrast, the LV outflow tract is bordered by the anterior (or septal) mitral leaflet, since the semilunar annulus is in fibrous continuity with the mitral annulus as demonstrated in Figures 30-1 and 30-2.

EXCEPTION

In double outlet right ventricle (DORV) there is no arterial outlet from the LV; therefore, characterization of the outflow tract will not aid in identification of the LV.

PART IV. Conotruncal Abnormalities

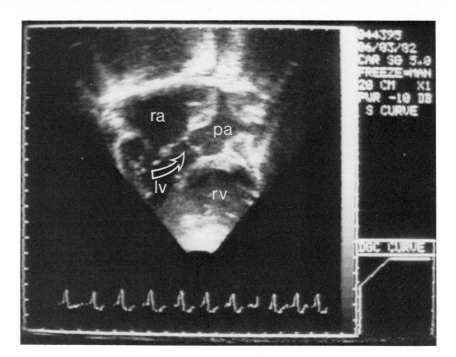

Fig. 30-2. Apical long-axis view of the left ventricle (*lv*) of patient with corrected transposition of the great arteries. The right atrium (*ra*) connects with the right-sided, morphologic lv via the mitral valve. The lv outflow tract is indicated by the arrow. The septal or medial mitral leaflet forms the right border of the left ventricular outflow. The pulmonary annulus is continuous with the mitral annulus. The pulmonary artery (*pa*) rises from the lv. An oblique view of the right ventricle (*rv*) is obtained from this view. The tricuspid valve is not seen.

Fig. 30-3. Parasternal long-axis view of the right ventricle (*rv*) in corrected transposition of the great arteries shows the alignment of the aorta (*ao*) with the rv and the separation of the annuli of the aorta and tricuspid valves (*arrows*) by conus muscle. *la* = left atrium.

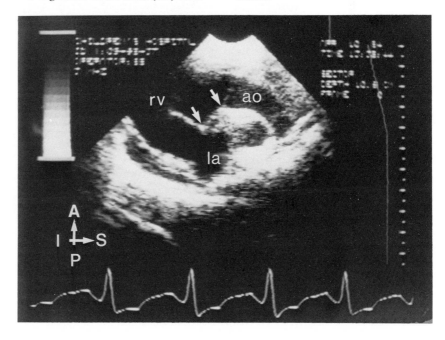

Trabecular and Papillary Muscle Pattern

1. The RV has a single large papillary muscle arising from the septomodera-ter band near its point of separation from the septal surface. The LV has two papillary muscles attached only to the free wall (Fig. 30-4).

   EXCEPTION

   In parachute mitral valve deformity, there is a single or two closely spaced papillary muscles within the LV. Nonetheless, each papillary muscle attaches only to the free wall.

2. The trabecular pattern of the right septal surface is coarser than that of the left.

   EXCEPTION

   Sometimes the differences in trabecular pattern are too subtle to distinguish, particularly when there is extreme RV dilation.

Ventricular Shape

The normal RV has the appearance of a cylinder (infundibulum) on top of a trapezoid (RV sinus), whereas the LV is shaped like a prolate ellipsoid.

EXCEPTIONS

1. The infundibulum is rarely dissociated from the RV sinus.
2. Ventricular shape is at least partly determined by the relative volume and/or pressure loads. Therefore, factors like interventricular curvature cannot be considered reliable indicators of ventricular morphology.

Fig. 30-4. A short-axis view of the left ventricle (*LV*) shows the morphology of the two free-wall papillary muscles in the LV. The right-left positions of the ventricles are reversed. *IVS* = interventricular septum; *RV* = right ventricle.

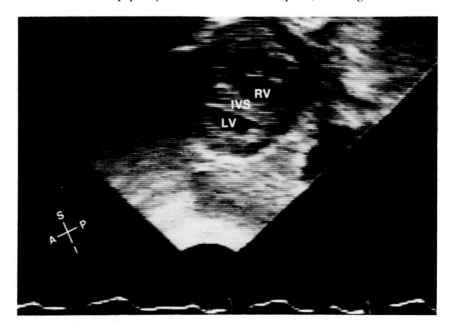

Great Artery Position

The loop rule states that the RV and aorta are usually on the same side. Therefore, the right-left relationship of the great arteries indicates the ventricular loop.

EXCEPTION

Exceptions to this rule are relatively common, however, so that this is a supportive, not a diagnostic, finding.

As one can see, there is an exception to almost every characteristic of ventricular morphology that has been used in ventricular identification. Therefore, all features must be considered when determining the ventricular identity.

Hand Rule

The hand rule states that just as a glove may be characterized as right- or left-handed, irrespective of the position from which it is viewed, so may the ventricular morphology be characterized, depending on whether the ventricular looping is normal (d-ventricular) or inverted (l-ventricular). Portions of the RV are related to the anatomy of the hand (Fig. 30-5A, B): the thumb to the tricuspid valve, the RV outflow tract to the fingers, the palm to the IVS, and the back of the hand to the RV free wall. If these components match the right hand, it is a d-ventricular loop; if they match the left hand, an l-ventricular loop. This rule is particularly useful when the ventricles are related in a direct anteroposterior (A-P) or superoinferior manner.

Fig. 30-5. Drawings depict chirality, or handedness, of the right ventricle (*RV*) as a means of defining ventricular situs. (A) The normal relations of RV structures. The thumb represents RV inflow; the fingers, RV outflow; the palm, the interventricular septum; and the back of the hand, the RV free wall. These relations are reversed in (B), which displays these relations of the RV with ventricular inversion. *RPA* = right pulmonary artery.

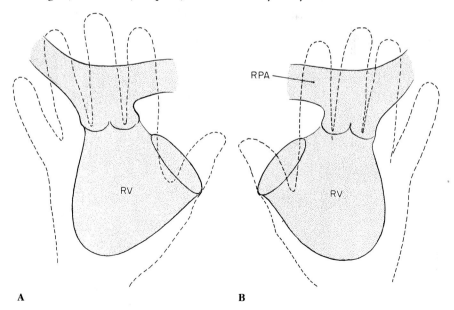

A   B

Echocardiographically, these relationships must be determined by sub-xiphoid or parasternal short-axis sweeps, while carefully noting the right-left coordinates of the tricuspid valve and the RV outflow tract and relating them to the position of the transducer. Alternatively, once the positions of the RV septal and free-wall surfaces are noted, the tricuspid valve and RV outflow tract can be demonstrated in a single plane. The right-left coordinates of the scan plane are then related to the right-left positions of the structures.

EXAMINATION
TECHNIQUE

Since the IVS is in a nearly sagittal plane, the transducer beam from a left parasternal position may not display the septum, but may only cross the free wall of the left-sided anatomic RV. In older patients, the right-sided anatomic LV may be obscured beneath the sternum. Nevertheless, positioning the patient in a steep left-lateral decubitus position will bring at least part of both ventricles into view. Short-axis views from this position are most helpful. In the younger child, subxiphoid short-axis sweeps provide a complete view of ventricular anatomy.

The apical and subxiphoid 4-chamber views demonstrate the level of attachment of the A-V valves.

Subxiphoid and suprasternal views demonstrate the position, origin, and branching pattern of the great arteries. The A-P and right-left positions of the great arteries can be seen from the parasternal short-axis position.

PROBLEMS

The echocardiographic diagnosis of simple L-TGA is not difficult because there are so many criteria that may be used to determine ventricular morphology. Because each of these criteria has notable exceptions in complex C-TGA, all possible clues must be used, and this is only possible when there is an adequate acoustic window to view ventricular inflow and outflow areas.

BIBLIOGRAPHY

Aziz, K. U., Paul, M., and Muster, A. J. Echocardiographic assessment of the left ventricular outflow tract in D-transposition of the great artery. *Am. J. Cardiol.* 41:543, 1978.

Coez, J. L., Ravault, M. C., and Worms, A. M. Complete atrioventricular canal defect associated with congenitally corrected transposition of the great arteries: Two-dimensional echocardiographic identification. *J. Am. Coll. Cardiol.* 1:1123, 1983.

Foale, R., Stefanini, L., Rickaids, A., et al. Left and right ventricular morphology in complex congenital heart disease by two-dimensional echocardiography. *Am. J. Cardiol.* 49:93, 1982.

Sutherland, G. R., Smallhorn, J. F., Anderson, R. H., et al. Atrioventricular discordance cross-sectional echocardiographic-morphologic correlative study. *Br. Heart J.* 50:8, 1983.

Trowitzsch, E., Colan, S. D., and Sanders, S. P. Two-dimensional echocardiographic estimation of right ventricular area change and ejection fraction in infants within systemic right ventricle. (Transposition of the great arteries or hypoplastic left heart syndrome.) *Am. J. Cardiol.* 55:1153, 1985.

PART IV. Conotruncal Abnormalities

Van Praagh, R., David, I., Wright, G. B., and Van Praagh, S. Ventricular Diagnosis and Designation. In M. J. Goodman (ed.), *Pediatric Cardiology*. Edinburgh and London: Churchill Livingstone, 1982. Pp. 153–168.

Van Praagh, R., Van Praagh, S., Vlad, K., and Keith, J. D. Anatomic types of congenital dextrocardia: Diagnostic and embryologic implications. *Am. J. Cardiol.* 13:510, 1964.

Van Praagh, R., Weinberg, P. M., Matsuoka, R., and Van Praagh, S. Malpositions of the Heart. In F. H. Adams and G. Emmanualides (eds.), *Moss' Heart Disease in Infants, Children and Adolescents*. Baltimore and London: Williams & Wilkins, 1983. Pp. 422–457.

CHAPTER 30. Corrected or L-Transposition of the Great Arteries

Double Outlet Right Ventricle

ANATOMY

Double outlet right ventricle (DORV) is an extremely heterogeneous category of anomalies with one common feature: Both great arteries are aligned with the right ventricle (RV). Currently, there is no universally accepted definition of DORV. To some, this term means origin of one great artery and at least 50 percent of the other over the RV; others require the presence of conus muscle between both great arteries and the atrioventricular (A-V) annulus. To avoid ambiguity, the following descriptions will refer to cases in which both criteria are fulfilled.

Since DORV is associated with a normal ventricular (d-ventricular) loop in the majority of patients, DORV will imply d-ventricular loop in this chapter, unless otherwise specified. In DORV, the great arteries are located entirely or almost entirely over the right ventricular sinus or infundibulum. One or both great arteries may arise from an infundibular chamber. The amount of subarterial conus muscle may vary considerably. Hence, the semilunar valves may lie (1) side by side, (2) with the pulmonary valve more anterior and superior (the tetralogy-of-Fallot type of DORV), or (3) with a more anterior and superior aortic valve (the transposition type of DORV) (Fig. 31-1A, B, C). Only subpulmonary conus muscle is seen in most cases of DORV with mitral atresia.

The infundibular (outflow) septum extends inferiorly between the pulmonary and aortic annuli. Its position is quite variable and may obstruct pulmonary or aortic outflow. Either outflow area may be further narrowed by hypoplasia of the conus free wall or abnormal A-V valve attachments. Size discrepancy between the two great arteries strongly suggests the presence of obstruction beneath the smaller of the two; alternatively, both outflows may be entirely unobstructed.

Fig. 31-1. (A) Drawing shows double outlet right ventricle (*RV*) with side-by-side great arteries. The semilunar valves are at approximately the same level. The infundibular septum lies in a straight sagittal plane. The ventricular septal defect (*VSD*) is subpulmonary. (B) Drawing of tetralogy-of-Fallot type of double outlet RV. Although both great arteries arise from the RV, the pulmonary artery (*PA*) is the more anterior and superior of the two. The infundibular septum is shifted to the left, narrowing the subpulmonary area. The VSD is subaortic, and the aorta (*Ao*) partially overrides the septum. This lesion is very similar to tetralogy of Fallot, except that the aorta is slightly more anterior and there is discontinuity between the aorta and mitral valve. (C) Drawing of transposition type of double outlet RV. The aorta is anterior and superior to the PA. The rightward shift of the infundibular septum may cause subaortic obstruction, in which case, there may be other downstream obstructive lesions such as coarctation or interruption of the aortic arch. The VSD is subpulmonic. The PA, which may override the septum to some degree, is slightly more anterior than in transposition of the great arteries. Also, unlike transposition of the great arteries, there is pulmonary-mitral discontinuity. *LV* = left ventricle.

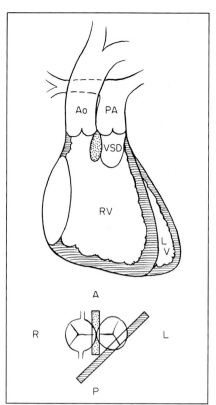

A

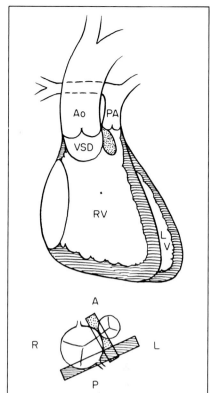

B

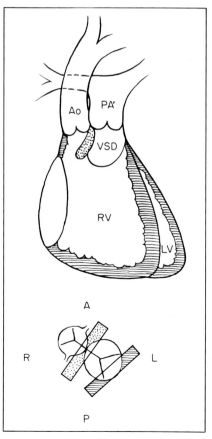

C

Fig. 31-3. Subxiphoid long-axis view angulated superiorly to a coronal section of right ventricle shows a common A-V valve anomaly in the double outlet right ventricle. The tricuspid valve (*TV*) is attached to the displaced infundibular septum (*arrow*) in addition to its attachments to the trabecular septum. *AO* = aortic root; *LV* = left ventricle; *PA* = pulmonary artery.

EXAMINATION TECHNIQUE

The relative anteroposterior (A-P) positions of the great arteries can be determined from a parasternal short-axis view. The parasternal long-axis view demonstrates the position of the more posterior semilunar root in relation to the IVS and anterior mitral leaflet and is an excellent view for determining the presence of subarterial conus muscle.

The subxiphoid views demonstrate the position of both great arteries over the ventricles by simultaneous display of the long axes of both great arteries and ventricles from multiple planes. When the great arteries are side by side, a coronal plane of the RV from a superiorly angulated long-axis (L4) transducer position displays the vessels simultaneously (Fig. 31-3). If the aorta is more anterior, the transducer must be rotated clockwise, the equivalent of a left anterior oblique angiographic projection, in order to display both great arteries. If the pulmonary artery (PA) is more anterior, the transducer is rotated counterclockwise, equivalent to a right-anterior oblique angiographic projection. This description applies only to D-malposed great arteries in which the aortic valve is rightward of the pulmonary valve.

Each great artery is displayed on standard long- and short-axis subxiphoid sweeps. When the transducer is rotated until both great vessels are seen simultaneously, the position of the transducer will indicate the relative positions of the great arteries and will display the infundibular or outflow septum. Unlike standard sweeping techniques, one finds the correct view and then notes the transducer position.

PROBLEMS

Two key features of DORV, bilateral subarterial conus muscle and origin of the great arteries from the RV, present diagnostic problems. A small subarterial conus muscle may be difficult to recognize; the resulting displacement of the posterior semilunar root may be minor. Moreover, an attenuated intervalvular fibrosa without interposed conus muscle may also be associated with slight anterior displacement of the semilunar root relative to the anterior mitral leaflet. Determination of the presence or absence of semilunar−A-V discontinuity may be subtle in these cases.

The degree of overriding of a semilunar root may also be difficult to ascertain. Tangential views through the root may create a false impression of its position relative to the IVS. Also, the IVS may be curved. Therefore, this relation must be determined by careful sweeps for multiple transducer positions. If different views do not coincide, the position of the great artery should be termed "ambiguous."

The most important source of error is related not to imaging, but to inconsistent use of nomenclature. In reporting these complex anomalies, it is more important to state each component anatomic feature (positions of great arteries, VSD, and so on) than to assign the lesion to an arbitary conoventricular type.

BIBLIOGRAPHY

DiSessa, T. G., Hagan, A. D., Pope, C., et al. Two-dimensional echocardiographic characteristics of double outlet right ventricle. *Am. J. Cardiol.* 44:1146, 1979.

Hagler, D. J., Abdul, J. T., Seward, J. B., Mair, D. D., and Ritter, D. G. Double outlet right ventricle wide angle two dimensional echocardiographic observation. *Circulation* 63:419, 1981.

Lev, M., and Bharati, S. Double outlet right ventricle. Association with other cardiovascular anomalies. *Arch. Pathol.* 95:117, 1973.

Van Praagh, S., Davidoff, A., Chin, A., et al. Double outlet right ventricle: Anatomic types and developmental implications based on a study of 101 autopsied cases. *Coeur* 13, 1982.

CHAPTER 31. Double Outlet Right Ventricle

Truncus Arteriosus

ANATOMY

In truncus arteriosus, a single arterial root arises above the ventricular chambers to supply the coronary, pulmonary, and systemic circulations, in that order. The truncal valve may override the interventricular septum (IVS) or arise directly over the right or left ventricle (RV and LV, respectively). There is usually a large malalignment subtruncal ventricular septal defect (VSD), although in rare circumstances this defect may be small or absent. The truncal valve is usually abnormal, with two to six thickened, myxomatous cusps. There is no connection between the RV and pulmonary arteries (PAs). The main pulmonary artery (MPA) may arise from the lateral or posterior border of the truncus (type 1); the branch PAs may arise separately from the back or sides of the truncal root (type 2); rarely, one of the branch PAs may be absent (type 3); finally, the truncus may be associated with interrupted aortic arch (type 4). In type 4, the truncal root divides into a small ascending aortic component that supplies some or all of the brachiocephalic arteries. The descending aorta and any brachiocephalic arteries not supplied from the ascending aorta are perfused from the large MPA via the ductus arteriosus. The origins of the PAs may be stenotic, but more commonly are widely patent, allowing a large pulmonary bloodflow. As a result, the left atrium (LA) and LV are usually dilated.

DIAGNOSTIC ECHO
FINDINGS

Documentation of the origin of PAs as they arise separately or via a single trunk from the ascending portion of a single arterial root is the requisite finding for this diagnosis (Fig. 32-1A, B).

The single arterial trunk usually overrides the IVS. A malalignment type of VSD is present as in tetralogy of Fallot. In rare variations, the arterial root may lie completely over the RV or LV.

No RV outflow tract is visualized in this lesion.

EXAMINATION
TECHNIQUE

If the PAs arise from the left side of the truncal root, they may be demonstrated by a view that shows right and left coordinates, such as a coronal suprasternal or subxiphoid (L3−4) or short-axis parasternal view. If the PAs arise from the back of the truncal root, then a view showing its anteroposterior (A-P) coordinates, such as a subxiphoid short-axis or parasternal long- or short-axis view, should be used.

The relationship of the truncal root to the IVS and ventricles below may be best seen on parasternal or apical long-axis or subxiphoid (S3) short-axis views that demonstrate the superoinferior coordinates of ventricular outflow.

Fig. 32-1. (A) Arteriogram of a patient with truncus arteriosus. In this case, the main pulmonary artery (*mpa*) arises from the left side of the common truncal root. (B) Echocardiogram from the same patient, obtained from a subxiphoid long-axis (L3) transducer position. The pulmonary arteries arise from a single trunk (*mpa*) on the left side of the common truncus (*ct*). The branch pulmonary arteries (not seen) are displayed by angling the transducer slightly posteriorly from this view. *asc ao* = ascending aorta; *lv* = left ventricle; *ra* = right atrium; *rv* = right ventricle.

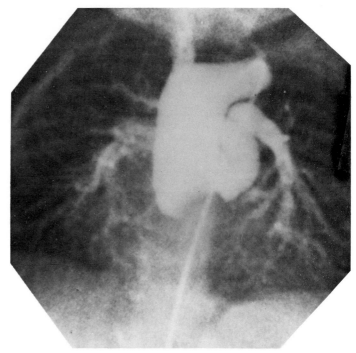

A

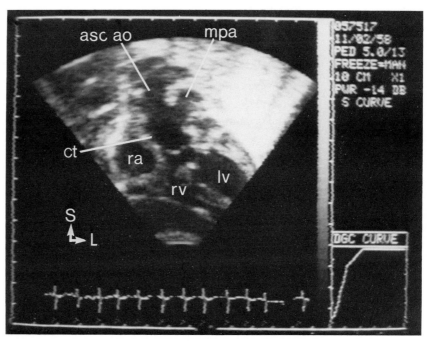

B

CHAPTER 32. Truncus Arteriosus

Fig. 32-2. Subxiphoid long-axis view (L3) in a patient with truncus arteriosus and interrupted aortic arch. Note the large pulmonary artery segment and small ascending aorta (*Asc Ao*), the reverse of the proportion shown in Figure 31-1A, B. Also, no transverse aortic arch can be seen from any view as the ascending aorta ends at the left carotid branch. *CT* = common truncus; *MPA* = main pulmonary artery; *RA* = right atrium; *RV* = right ventricle.

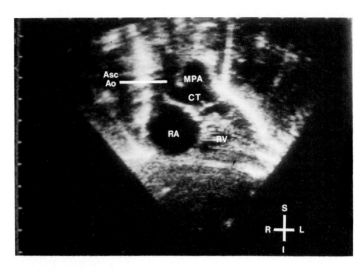

ASSOCIATED LESIONS

In the neonate, truncus arteriosus can be associated with interrupted aortic arch. The MPA segment coming off the truncal root is quite large, while the arterial portion continuing to the aortic arch is proportionally smaller (Fig. 32-2). This finding should strongly suggest the associated interrupted aortic arch.

Truncus arteriosus may be associated with a complete atrioventricular (A-V) canal.

PROBLEMS

If the origin of the PAs cannot be visualized, the diagnosis of truncus arteriosus may be confused with tetralogy of Fallot with pulmonary atresia. In both lesions, there is a large semilunar root overriding a VSD, and there may be no demonstrable RV outflow tract. Therefore, it is imperative to identify the origin of the PAs properly in order to make the specific diagnosis.

BIBLIOGRAPHY

Barron, J. V., Sahn, D. J., Attie, F., et al. Two dimensional echocardiographic study of right ventricular outflow anatomy in pulmonary atresia with ventricular septal defect and in truncus arteriosus. *Am. Heart J.* 105:281, 1983.

Frary, G., Albers, W., and Shah, J. Echocardiographic findings of isolated anomalous origin of the right pulmonary artery from the ascending aorta. *J. Cardiovasc. Ultrasonogr.* 2:285, 1983.

Gerlis, L. M., Wilson, N., Dickinson, D. F., et al. Valvar stenosis in truncus arteriosus. *Br. Heart J.* 52:440, 1984.

Houston, A. B., Gregory, N. L., Montaugh, I. L., et al. Two dimensional echocardiography in infants with persistent truncus arteriosus. *Br. Heart J.* 46:492, 1981.

Rice, M. J., Seward, J. B., Hagler, D. J., et al. Definitive diagnosis of truncus arteriosus by two-dimensional echocardiography. *Mayo Clin. Proc.* 57:467, 1982.

Riggs, T. W., and Paul, M. H. Two dimensional echocardiographic prospective diagnosis of common truncus arteriosus in infants. *Am. J. Cardiol.* 50:1380, 1982.

Smallhorn, J. F., Anderson, R. H., and Macartney, F. J. Two-dimensional echocardiographic assessment of communications between ascending aorta and pulmonary trunk or individual pulmonary arteries. *Br. Heart J.* 47:563, 1982.

Complex Heart Disease

Sanders, S. P. Echocardiography and related techniques in the diagnosis of congenital heart defects. Part II: Atrioventricular valves and ventricles. *Echocardiography* 1:333, 1984.

Sanders, S. P. Echocardiography and related techniques in the diagnosis of congenital heart defects. Part III: Conotruncus and great arteries. *Echocardiography* 1:443, 1984.

Snider, A. R., Ports, T. A., and Silverman, N. H. Venous anomalies of the coronary sinus: Detection by M-mode, two-dimensional and contrast echocardiography. *Circulation* 60:721, 1979.

PART V. Complex Heart Disease

Single Ventricle

ANATOMY

Although terminology is currently changing, the term *single ventricle* will be used here to describe the family of complex lesions in which a single ventricular chamber receives blood from both atria via two separate or a single common atrioventricular (A-V) valve. Tricuspid and mitral atresias are discussed separately in Chapters 14 and 20. Straddling A-V valves are discussed in Chapter 35.

Most single ventricles are of left ventricular (LV) morphology or have characteristics of both ventricles (common ventricles). The single LV is associated with an anterior outflow chamber (also considered a hypoplastic ventricle) that is positioned to the right (d-ventricular loop) or left (l-ventricular loop) of the larger posterior LV (Fig. 34-1A to C). Commonly, the aorta arises from the anterior outflow chamber, in which case it is vulnerable to subaortic obstruction at the opening of this chamber into the larger LV chamber. This opening is variously called the *bulboventricular foramen*, or a ventricular septal defect (VSD). Subaortic obstruction at this site is often associated with coarctation of the aorta or interrupted aortic arch. An uncommon but interesting form of single ventricle, known as Holmes's heart, is a double inlet single LV with normally interrelated great arteries and a subpulmonary infundibular chamber. Some degree of infundibular pulmonary stenosis is usually present. The physiology and conotruncal anatomy are similar to tetralogy of Fallot.

Single RV is rare and is usually associated with a posterior hypoplastic LV (or trabecular pouch) that has no inflow or outflow tract.

DIAGNOSTIC ECHO
FINDINGS

Regardless of terminology used, the following anatomic features must be clearly defined:

1. Positions of atria
2. Position of atrial septum relative to A-V valves
3. Number, position, and attachment of A-V valves relative to the larger ventricular sinus and hypoplastic ventricle (outflow chamber)
4. Size of the communication between the ventricular chambers (bulboventricular foramen or VSD)
5. Presence and right-left position of the outflow chamber relative to the larger ventricular chamber, or if no anterior chamber is present, presence and position of a posterior pouch or hypoplastic LV
6. Origin and position of both great arteries

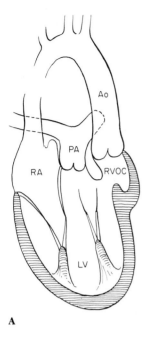

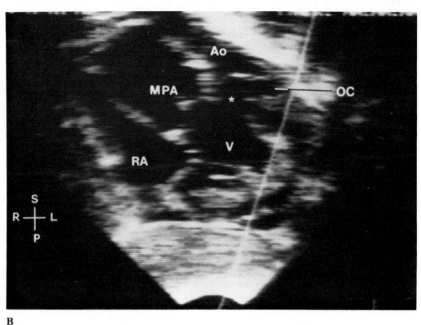

A

B

Fig. 34-1. (A) Drawing of double inlet single left ventricle (*LV*) with l-ventricular loop. The right ventricular outflow chamber (*RVOC*) is anterior and to the left of the larger left ventricular chamber and gives rise to a leftward-placed aorta (*Ao*). The pulmonary root is posterior, inferior, and to the right of the aortic annulus and arises directly from the left ventricular chamber. (B) Subxiphoid long-axis view with clockwise rotation, similar to that shown in Figure 34-1A, in a patient with single ventricle (*V*) with L-transposition of the great arteries. A di-lated main pulmonary artery (*MPA*) rises from the larger ventricular chamber. The leftward aorta is smaller than the pulmonary artery and arises from a leftward, superior, and anterior outflow chamber (*OC*) with a narrowed orifice (*star*). (C) Long-axis view with extreme anterior angulation in a patient with single ventricle and L-transposition of the great arteries similar to that shown in Figure 34-1B. Again, the orifice (*star*) of the right ventricular outflow tract (*RVOT*) is narrow. *Asc. Aorta* = ascending aorta; *PA* = pulmonary artery; *RA* = right atrium.

EXAMINATION
TECHNIQUES

The examination (in levocardia) is performed as usual. Subxiphoid (L1 and L2) views are useful for detecting the atrial situs and the presence and size of an interatrial communication. Subxiphoid or apical 4-chamber views are used to determine the number and size of A-V valves (Fig. 34-2A, B). The posterior semilunar root is seen by angling anteriorly from the 4-chamber view and is located between the two A-V valves (Fig. 34-3A, B). Fibrous continuity between the posterior root and both A-V valves is the rule. Subpulmonary stenosis, due to endocardial cushion tissue, may be present. The anterior outflow chamber and the anterior semilunar root are best seen by further anterior angulation (L4, L5). Depending on the ventricular loop, the outflow chamber will be left-sided (l-ventricular loop) or right-sided (d-ventricular loop). The size of the bulboventricular foramen should be noted in two planes.

PART V. Complex Heart Disease

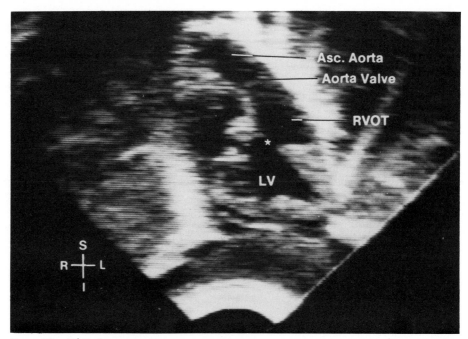

C   **Fig. 34-1.** (continued)

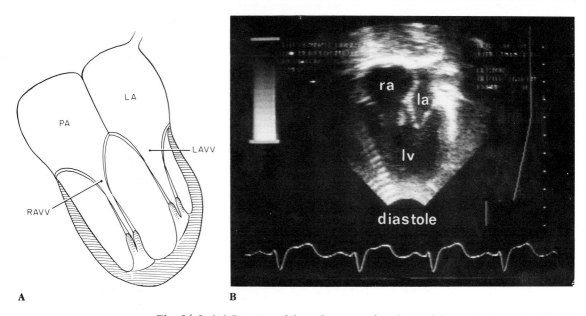

A   B

Fig. 34-2. (A) Drawing of the inflow portion of a double inlet single ventricle shows two separate atrioventricular valves providing outflow from the right and left atria into a single ventricular chamber. The atrioventricular valves attach to papillary muscles in the floor of the left ventricle. This view may be obtained from apical or subxiphoid 4-chamber views. (B) Companion echo shows apical long-axis view in a patient with double inlet single left ventricle. *LA, la* = left atrium; *LAVV* = left atrioventricular valve; *lv* = left ventricle; *PA* = pulmonary artery; *ra* = right atrium; *RAVV* = right atrioventricular valve.

CHAPTER 34. Single Ventricle

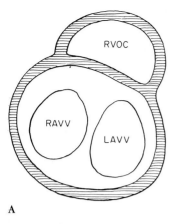

A

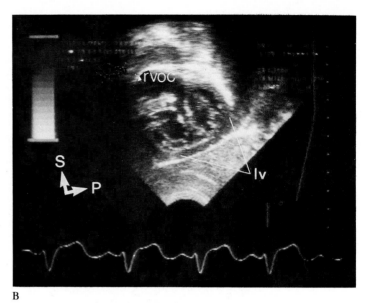

B

Fig. 34-3. Drawing (A) and echo (B) of subxiphoid short-axis view in the same patient show cross sections of the atrioventricular valve orifices. *LAVV* = left atrioventricular valve; *lv* = left ventricle; *RAVV* = right atrioventricular valve; *RVOC, rvoc* = right ventricular outflow chamber.

Subxiphoid or parasternal short-axis views are useful for detecting the morphology of the ventricle and A-V valves and for assessing the size of the bulboventricular foramen in a plane orthogonal to the long-axis plane (Fig. 34-3A, B). The pulmonary artery (PA) anatomy can be determined in the subxiphoid long-axis or parasternal high transverse views. The aortic arch should be evaluated in a transverse subxiphoid or suprasternal notch (SSN) view because coarctation or interrupted aortic arch is common in the setting of a restrictive bulboventricular foramen.

Technique for examining complex lesions in dextrocardia cannot be prescribed. Views must be designed to fit the circumstances. Again, careful documentation of the scan planes is essential for viewing the echocardiograms in the future.

BIBLIOGRAPHY

Anton, R. T., Becker, A. E., Moller, J. H., et al. Double inlet left ventricle: Straddling tricuspid valve. *Br. Heart J.* 36:747, 1974.

Beardshaw, J. A., Gibson, D. G., Pearson, M. C., et al. Echocardiographic diagnosis of primitive ventricle with two atrioventricular valves. *Br. Heart J.* 39:266, 1977.

Bharati, S., McAllister, H. A., and Lev, M. Straddling and displaced atrioventricular orifices and valves. *Circulation* 60:673, 1979.

Freedom, R. M., Picchio, F., Duncan, W. J., et al. The atrioventricular junction in the univentricular heart: A two dimensional echocardiographic analysis. *Pediatr. Cardiol.* 3:105, 1982.

Perez-Martinez, V. M., Garcia-Fernandez, F., Oliver-Ruiz, J., et al. Double-outlet right atrium with two atrioventricular valves and left atrial outlet atresia. *J. Am. Coll. Cardiol.* 3:375, 1984.

Rigby, M. L., Anderson, R. H., Gibson, D., et al. Two-dimensional echocardiographic categorization of the univentricular heart: Ventricular morphology, type and mode of atrioventricular connection. *Br. Heart J.* 46:603, 1981.

Sahn, D. J., Harder, J. R., Freedom, R. M., et al. Cross-sectional echocardiographic diagnosis and subclassification of univentricular hearts: Imaging studies of atrio-ventricular valves, septal structures and rudimentary outflow chambers. *Circulation* 66:1070, 1982.

Seward, J. B., Tajik, A. J., Hagler, D. J., et al. Echocardiogram and common (single) ventricle: Angiographic-anatomic correlation. *Am. J. Cardiol.* 39:217, 1977.

Smallhorn, J. F., Tommasini, G., and Macartney, F. J. Two dimensional echocardio-graphic assessment of common atrioventricular valves in univentricular hearts. *Br. Heart J.* 46:30, 1981.

Van Praagh, R., Plett, J. A., Van Praagh, S. Single ventricle. Pathology, embryology, terminology and classification. *Herz* 4:113, 1979.

Van Praagh, R., Van Praagh, S., Vlad, P., et al. Diagnosis of the anatomic types of single or common ventricle. *Am. J. Cardiol.* 15:345, 1965.

Straddling Atrioventricular Valves

Either tricuspid or mitral valves may straddle the interventricular septum (IVS). In such cases, it is important to describe the entire atrioventricular (A-V) valve apparatus in relation to the IVS. The annulus overrides the septum through a ventricular septal defect (VSD). The A-V valve is described as straddling the IVS when it has attachments on both sides of the IVS in both ventricles.

Tricuspid valves virtually always straddle through an A-V canal (inlet) VSD (Figs. 35-1A to C, 35-2A, B). The septal tricuspid leaflet may be attached to the left side of the IVS or to a papillary muscle within the left ventricle (LV). The inflow portion of the right ventricle (RV) may be hypoplastic, in proportion to the degree that the tricuspid valve overrides into the LV. The relationship of the straddling tricuspid valve to the IVS is best displayed from the apical and subxiphoid 4-chamber views when these views show the chordae and their attachments within both ventricles. The subxiphoid short-axis scan displays chordal attachments of the septal tricuspid leaflet.

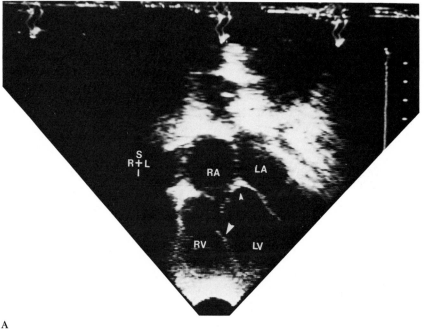

A

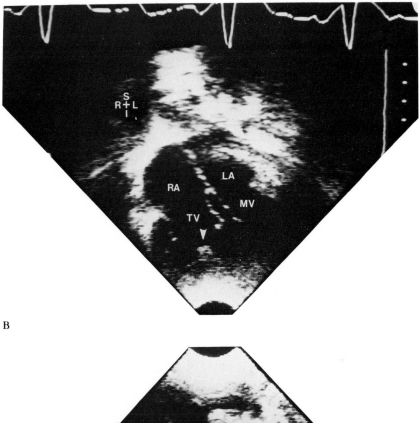

B

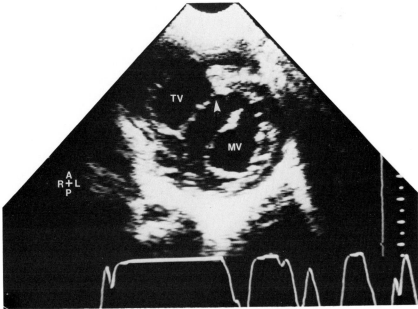

C

Fig. 35-1. (A) Systolic frame of a 4-chamber view of patient with overriding tricuspid valve. The cardiac crux, the junction between the lower border of the interatrial septum and the annuli of the tricuspid and mitral valves (*small arrow*) is displaced to left of the trabecular muscular interventricular septum (*large arrow*). In addition, the coaptation point of the tricuspid leaflets is immediately above the interventricular septum. The right ventricle (*RV*) is smaller than the left ventricle (*LV*). (B) Diastolic frame of the same patient. The arrow indicates the crest of the trabecular muscular septum. (C) Parasternal short-axis view of the same patient shows the cross section of the tricuspid orifice within the ventricular septal defect attached to the left septal surface (*arrow*). *LA* = left atrium; *MV* = mitral valve; *RA* = right atrium; *TV* = tricuspid valve.

Fig. 35-2. (A) Subxiphoid long-axis view shows the central fibrous body (*arrow*) displaced over the left ventricle (*lv*).and a portion of the tricuspid valve entering the lv in a patient with straddling tricuspid valve. (B) Companion subxiphoid short-axis view in same patient. Note the similar appearance of straddling tricuspid valve (*tv*) and common atrioventricular canal. The small mitral valve (*mv*) can be seen in the more superior part of the left ventricle (*lv*). *rv* = right ventricle.

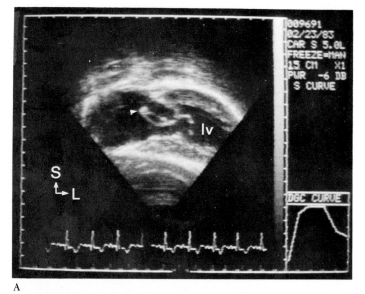

A

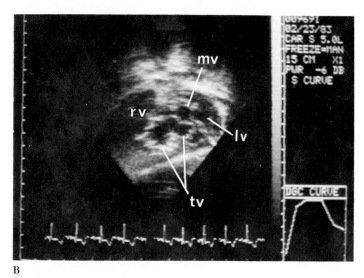

B

Fig. 35-3. Subxiphoid short-axis view in a patient with straddling mitral valve. The straddling portion of the mitral valve (*arrow*) crosses the septum through an anterior malalignment ventricular septal defect. The tricuspid valve is inferior to the lower margin of the ventricular septal. *lv* = left ventricle; *rv* = right ventricle.

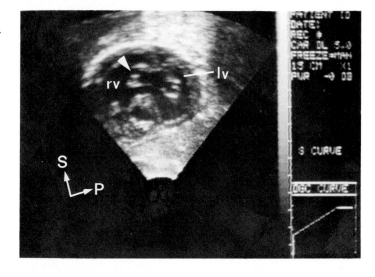

The straddling mitral valve communicates with the morphologic RV via a malalignment or outlet type of VSD. This defect is commonly associated with conotruncal abnormalities such as double outlet right ventricle (DORV) and transposition of the great arteries (TGA). This defect is often difficult to recognize because only a portion of the anterior leaflet of the A-V valve straddles the IVS, while the posterior portion of the valve attaches normally to the LV papillary muscles. The straddling portion of the valve usually attaches to a papillary muscle within the infundibulum. The superior portion of the trabecular IVS curves leftward to underride the mitral orifice. Because the lower septum is in a normal position, this gives the septum a hockey-stick configuration. The straddling mitral valve is best viewed from a subxiphoid or high parasternal short-axis view (Fig. 35-3). In general, any view clearly demonstrating the outflow septum will show the overriding portion of the anterior mitral leaflet and its connection, if any, to the outflow septum. The mitral valve may appear relatively normal from apical and subxiphoid 4-chamber views because these display the normally attached posterior portions of the valve leaflets. Anterior angulation from the apical 4-chamber view shows the straddling portion of the valve. The unusual hockey-stick configuration of the IVS is difficult to display in any one plane. The position of the septum will appear normal from an apical or subxiphoid 4-chamber view, but on anterior angulation, the septum will suddenly appear at a 90° angle, as if it were viewed from a short-axis position. Although this finding is only recognized by careful sweeping of the transducer, it is highly characteristic of overriding mitral valve, and its presence should prompt a careful survey of all mitral attachments.

The position of the line of coaptation A-V valve leaflets (systolic position) as well as all distal leaflet attachments must be described. Since a normally attached septal tricuspid leaflet may open into the LV outflow tract through an inlet or A-V canal VSD, the diastolic position of a valve should not be considered diagnostic of a straddling A-V valve.

BIBLIOGRAPHY

Bharati, S., McAllister, H. A., and Lev, M. Straddling and displaced atrioventricular orifices and valves. *Circulation* 60:673, 1979.

Muster, A. J., Bharati, S., Aziz, K. U., et al. Taussig-Bing anomaly with straddling mitral valve. *J. Thorac. Cardiovasc. Surg.* 77:832, 1979.

Rice, M. J., Seward, J. B., Edwards, W. D., et al. Straddling atrioventricular valve: Two-dimensional echocardiographic diagnosis, classification and surgical implications. *Am. J. Cardiol.* 55:505, 1985.

Seward, J. B., Tajik, A. J., and Ritter, D. G. Echocardiographic features of straddling tricuspid valve. *Mayo Clin. Proc.* 50:427, 1975.

Smallhorn, J. F., Tommasini, G., and Macartney, F. J. Detection and assessment of straddling and overriding atrioventricular valves by two-dimensional echocardiography. *Br. Heart J.* 46:254, 1981.

Tabry, I. F., McGoon, D. C., Danielson, G. K., et al. Surgical management of straddling atrioventricular valve. *J. Thorac. Cardiovasc. Surg.* 77:191, 1979.

Wenink, A. C. G., and DeGroot, A. C. G. Straddling mitral and tricuspid valves: Morphologic differences and developmental backgrounds. *Am. J. Cardiol.* 49:1959, 1982.

CHAPTER 35. Straddling Atrioventricular Valves

CHAPTER 36

Juxtaposition of the Atrial Appendages

NORMAL ANATOMY

The normal right atrial appendage (RAA) is a broad-based triangular structure rising anterior to the superior vena cava (SVC) and curving to the left to lie at the right border of the ascending aorta. The mouth of the RAA is best seen from a subxiphoid parasternal view demonstrating the long axis of the SVC as it enters the right atrium (RA) (Fig. 36-1). Sweeping slightly to the left from this position demonstrates the body of the RAA. Proceeding further leftward, the ascending aorta comes into view. The RAA may also be displayed from an anteriorly angulated subxiphoid long-axis view (L3 to L4) as an echo-free space to the right of the ascending aorta.

The origin of the left atrial appendage (LAA) lies close to the left pulmonary veins (PVs) and is often confused with them on echocardiographic examination. This base of the LAA is narrow, and the body is fingerlike. The appendage usually projects anteriorly to lie to the left of the pulmonary artery (PA). Its position is variable, however, and it can even project posteriorly. The LAA in its usual position can be displayed from a subxiphoid or apical 4-chamber view with slight counterclockwise rotation, a parasternal short-axis view, or a subxiphoid short-axis view (S4) that is just left of the right ventricular (RV) outflow tract and main pulmonary artery (MPA).

Fig. 36-1. Subxiphoid short-axis (S1) view demonstrates the long axis of the superior (*sup*) and inferior (*inf*) venae cavae in a normal heart. The broad-based mouth of the right atrial appendage (*RAA*) projects from the right atrial cavity anterior to the sup.

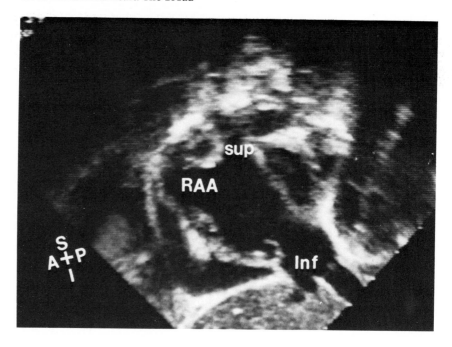

LEFT JUXTAPOSITION OF THE ATRIAL APPENDAGES
Anatomy

Left juxtaposition of the atrial appendages is commonly associated with other intracardiac anomalies, particularly transposition of the great arteries (TGA) and tricuspid atresia. The RAA, which communicates with the RA cavity, lies anterior and superior to LAA and directly behind the great arteries. This positioning affects the orientation of the interatrial septum: The superior portion of the interatrial septum (septum secundum) is deviated more posteriorly than normal, wrapping around in a curvilinear fashion to lie in a coronal plane. As a result, the RA cavity appears smaller than normal.

Fig. 36-2. (A) High transverse parasternal view in a patient with left juxtaposition of the atrial appendages. The right atrial appendage (*raa*) passes posterior to the posterior semilunar root and anterior to the left atrium (*la*). Note the curvilinear appearance of the interatrial septum. (B) Subxiphoid long-axis view shows the raa passing to the left in a plane just posterior to the posterior semilunar root. *ra* = right atrium.

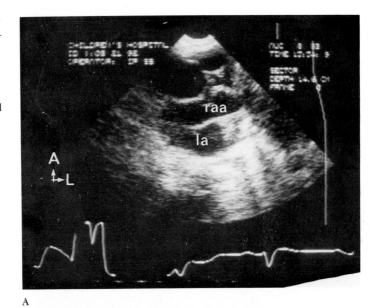

A

B

*Diagnostic Echo
Findings*

The presence of an abnormal septal orientation should prompt a careful evaluation of the position of the atrial appendages. Direct visualization of the atrial appendages posterior to and to the left of the great arteries is the most definitive finding for the diagnosis of left-juxtaposed atrial appendages.

*Examination
Techniques*

The juxtaposed atrial appendages may be displayed from a high parasternal short-axis view or an apical or subxiphoid 4-chamber view with anterior angulation (Fig. 36-2A, B). In parasternal short-axis view, the RAA can be seen passing to the left, posterior to the posterior semilunar root in a plane just superior to the semilunar valve. From the 4-chamber view, the RA appears small, and the posterior portion of the interatrial septum is seen. The RAA can be seen passing leftward in a plane just anterior to the atrioventricular (A-V) valves and just posterior to the semilunar root. The subxiphoid short-axis view of the midatrial cavity (S2) demonstrates posterior deviation of the septum secundum.

Problems

Recognition of the abnormal plane of the upper interatrial septum is a highly sensitive, but not entirely specific finding for left juxtaposition of the atrial appendages, since some cases with dextrocardia also have an abnormal atrial septal position in the absence of juxtaposed atrial appendage.

A long- or medium-long–focus transducer is required to visualize the atrial appendages from a subxiphoid or apical transducer position. Poor lateral resolution will cause overlap with other structures, such as PVs.

A left juxtaposed RAA may resemble a dilated coronary sinus in some views. However, the coronary sinus is a very posterior and inferior structure, while the juxtaposed atrial appendage is more superior and anterior to the left atrium (LA).

BIBLIOGRAPHY

Charuzi, Y., Spanos, P. K., Amplatz, K., et al. Juxtaposition of the atrial appendages. *Circulation* 47:620, 1973.

Chin, A. J., Bierman, F. Z., Williams, R. G., et al. Two-dimensional echocardiographic appearance of complete left-sided juxtaposition of the atrial appendages. *Am. J. Cardiol.* 52:346, 1983.

Rice, M. J., Seward, J. B., Hagler, D. J., et al. Left juxtaposed atrial appendages: Diagnostic two-dimensional echocardiographic features. *J. Am. Coll. Cardiol.* 1:1330, 1983.

Rosengart, G. C., Slark, J., and Taylor, J. F. N. Anatomical relationships in transposition of the great arteries: Juxtaposition of the atrial appendages. *Ann. Thorac. Surg.* 18:456, 1974.

CHAPTER 37

Cardiac Malpositions

The various standard echocardiographic views (i.e., precordial, apical, sub-xiphoid, and suprasternal notch [SSN]) described in Chapters 1 to 4, while valid for patients with levocardia, are of limited value for patients with cardiac malposition. The two basic goals for imaging such patients are (1) to determine the location and orientation of the heart, and (2) to devise sets of views that permit visualization of the heart in two or more planes. Since the planes of examination may be quite unusual (and unrecognizable at a future viewing), it is important to record the orientation of the transducer. A convenient method is to record a description of the transducer position using the audio channel of the videotape-recorder.

DEXTROCARDIA

In general, mirror images of the standard left chest views may be used effectively in dextrocardia. For a parasternal long-axis view, the transducer is placed in the third or fourth right intercostal space with the scan plane directed right-inferior and left-superior. For a parasternal short-axis view, the scan plane is directed right-superior and left-inferior. Subxiphoid long-axis views (Fig. 37-1) are obtained by angling the transducer superiorly and rightward, with some counterclockwise rotation about the long axis of the transducer. Subxiphoid short-axis views are obtained in the same manner as those for levocardia except that the transducer is angled to the right instead of the left.

Fig. 37-1. Subxiphoid long-axis view in a patient with dextrocardia. *la* = left atrium; *lv* = left ventricle; *ra* = right atrium.

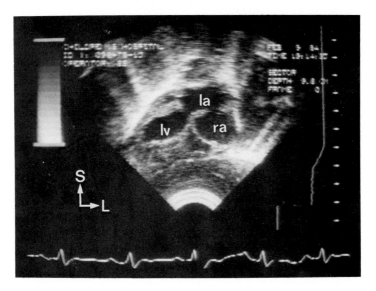

Fig. 37-2. Subxiphoid long-axis view in a patient with mesocardia. Note that mesocardia produces a foreshortened apical view because the apex of the heart points anteriorly and inferiorly. *lv* = left ventricle; *rv* = right ventricle.

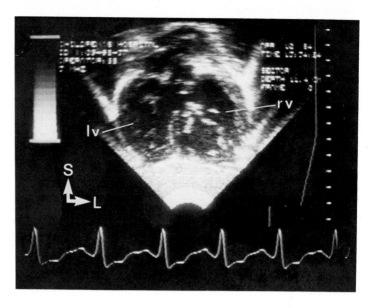

The left-right reversal of cardiac structure is obvious in long-axis and 4-chamber views. However, short-axis views may be indistinguishable from those obtained in levocardia because there may be no anteroposterior (A-P) inversion.

MESOCARDIA

Midline hearts are particularly difficult to examine. Their retrosternal position makes parasternal imaging difficult at best. Since the apex of the heart is positioned toward the subxiphoid space, orienting the transducer for subxiphoid long-axis views results in an apical 4-chamber view (Fig. 37-2). Attempts to obtain subxiphoid transverse views produce apical long-axis views of first one ventricle and then the other. True transverse views of the heart may be difficult to obtain. Rolling the patient to one side may allow the heart to move from behind the sternum far enough to obtain transverse parasternal views, with the transducer oriented in a transverse plane of the trunk (more clockwise rotation than usual for parasternal short-axis views).

BIBLIOGRAPHY

Huhta, J. C., Hagler, D. J., Seward, J. B., et al. Two dimensional echocardiographic assessment of dextrocardia: A segmental approach. *Am. J. Cardiol.* 50:1351, 1982.

Van Praagh, R., Van Praagh, S., Vlad, K., and Keith, J. D. Anatomic types of congenital dextrocardia: Diagnostic and embryologic implications. *Am. J. Cardiol.* 13:510, 1964.

Van Praagh, R., Weinberg, P. M., Matsuoka, R., and Van Praagh, S. Malpositions of the Heart. In F. H. Adams and G. Emmanualides (eds.), *Moss' Heart Disease in Infants, Children and Adolescents.* Baltimore and London: Williams & Wilkins, 1983. Pp. 422–457.

PART VI

Evaluation of Postoperative Patients

Evaluation of Postoperative Patients

Echocardiography can be of considerable value in evaluating patients following surgery. Early postoperative examination may be limited by residual mediastinal air, chest tubes, pacing wire, etc. However, with diligence, considerable information can be derived. If a left atrial (LA) catheter is available, contrast echocardiography is useful for detecting residual left-to-right shunts. Ventricular function may be determined by two-dimensional (2-D) echocardiography and 2-D derived M-mode. Also regional wall motion abnormalities suggestive of ischemia or infarction may be detected. Postoperative hemopericardium or pericardial effusion can be detected by 2-D echo. Doppler echocardiography is useful for detecting valve regurgitation, obstruction, and residual shunt lesions.

Prosthetic materials (Gortex, Dacron) used for patching intracardiac defects are extremely efficient reflectors. While easy to identify, patches cause shadowing or false dropout of subjacent structures. Thus, dropout near a patch should suggest a residual defect only if the echo beam has not first traversed the patch or if there is confirmation of shunting in the area by Doppler examination or contrast injection.

COMPLETE ATRIAL
SEPTAL
DEFECT REPAIR
Anatomy

Repair of common atrioventricular (A-V) canal involves patching of the ventricular septal defect (VSD), attachment (or suspension) of the A-V valves from the patch, and closure of the atrial septal defect (ASD) (using the same or separate patches for ASD and VSD). The cleft in the anterior mitral valve leaflet (division between the superior and inferior cushion components) may be sutured extensively or left divided, according to the judgment of the surgeon. In any case, the leaflets should coapt during systole. Postoperative complications that we have encountered include disruption of the atrial or ventricular portions of the patch and mitral regurgitation.

*Examination
Technique*

The ASD portion of the patch is best seen in subxiphoid 4-chamber and rightward short-axis views. The apical views can be used, but shadowing can be expected because of imaging through the patch.

The atrial portion of the patch should completely occupy the lower interatrial septum down to the level of the A-V valve (Fig. 38-1A, B). Disruption of the patch is usually due to failure of suture lines between the patch and interatrial septum. If disruption occurs, the patch material can usually be seen waving just above the intersection of the A-V valves (Fig. 38-2). An analogous picture is seen for disruption of the VSD portion of the patch—except that the defect and unattached portion of the patch are below the place of attachment of the A-V valve.

Fig. 38-1. Subxiphoid 4-chamber (A) and apical 4-chamber (B) views in a patient following a repair of complete A-V canal (septal) defect. The patch (*arrows*) can be seen connecting to the posterior interatrial septum and to the right side of the interventricular septum. *LA* = left atrium; *LV* = left ventricle; *RA* = right atrium; *RV* = right ventricle.

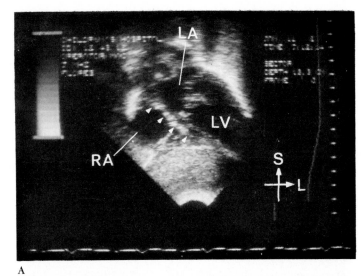

A

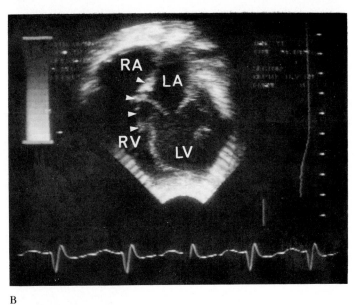

B

Fig. 38-2. Subxiphoid 4-chamber view in a patient with repaired complete atrioventricular septal defect and disruption of the interatrial portion of the patch. In real time, the edge of the patch (*arrow*) can be seen moving between right (*ra*) and left (*la*) atria during the cardiac cycle.

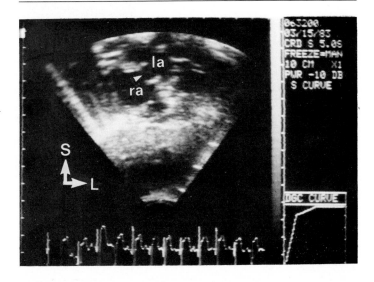

The mitral valve is best examined in subxiphoid L3, S3, and S4, apical 4-chamber, and parasternal long- and short-axis views (Fig. 38-3). The appearance of the valve is dependent on the surgical technique. If the cleft of the anterior mitral leaflet has been sutured, it moves as a single unit; if the cleft is not sutured, the superior and inferior cushion components move separately, giving the valve a tripartite appearance. Failure to demonstrate coaptation of the valve leaflets across the orifice in either a subxiphoid or parasternal short-axis scan is suggestive of mitral regurgitation. However, demonstration of leaflet coaptation across the orifice does not rule out mitral regurgitation. Doppler echocardiography is particularly helpful in evaluating mitral valve function.

VENTRICULAR SEPTAL DEFECT (INCLUDING TETRALOGY OF FALLOT) REPAIR
Anatomy

Repair of lesions including a VSD generally includes closure of the VSD with a Dacron or Gortex patch. The patch is sutured to the right septal surface, usually several millimeters from the edge of the defect, to avoid the conduction system. Obviously the location of the patch should correspond to the type of VSD. Associated procedures may include patch augmentation of the right ventricular (RV) outflow tract or interposition of a conduit between the RV and pulmonary artery (PA). The conduit may lie on either side of the aorta, depending on the position of the great arteries.

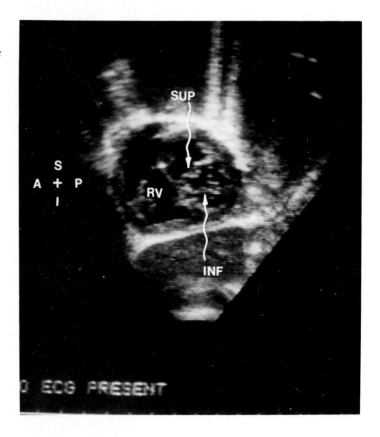

Fig. 38-3. Subxiphoid short-axis view (S4) in a patient with repaired complete atrioventricular septal defect. The superior (*SUP*) and inferior (*INF*) portions of the mitral valve are sutured to the septal defect patch. *RV* = right ventricle.

Examination Technique

The VSD is best seen in a subxiphoid or parasternal short-axis view of the appropriate area of the septum. The ventricular septal patch in tetralogy of Fallot is also well seen in a parasternal long-axis view (Fig. 38-4A, B). A residual VSD may result from disruption of sutures or improper placement of the patch. An edge of the patch may be sewn to a muscle bundle in the RV instead of the margin of the VSD (Fig. 38-5). In cases of double outlet right ventricle (DORV) or transposition of the great arteries (TGA) with VSD, it is possible to run the patch from the septal crest to the anterior RV free wall instead of the infundibular septum, creating a "no outlet right ventricle." The best clue to this potentially disastrous complication is the horizontal orientation of the patch seen in a subxiphoid short-axis view. Adequacy of the outflow tract RV patching is best seen in a precordial short-axis view.

Fig. 38-4. Subxiphoid long- (A) and short- (B) axis views in a patient with tetralogy of Fallot. The ventricular septal defect patch (*arrows*) appears as a bright linear echo between the anterior border of the aortic root (*Ao*) and the interventricular septum. *lv* = left ventricle; *ra* = right atrium; *rv* = right ventricle.

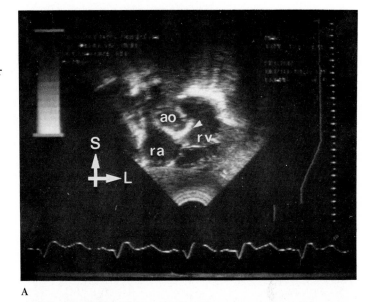

A

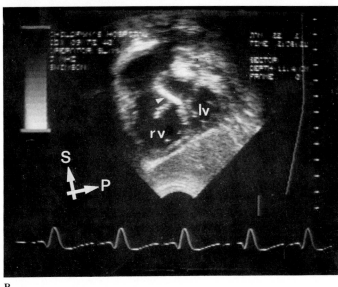

B

CHAPTER 38. Evaluation of Postoperative Patients

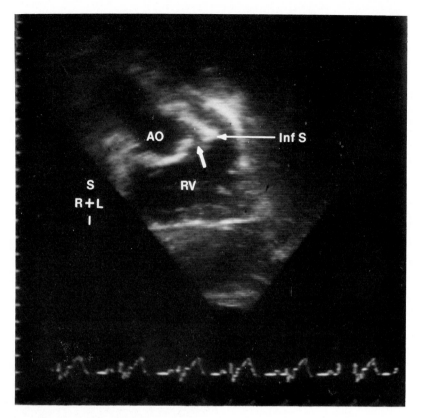

Fig. 38-5. Subxiphoid long-axis view with slight counterclockwise rotation in a patient with repaired tetralogy of Fallot. The bright echoes from the ventricular septal defect patch lie beneath the aorta (*AO*), excluding this vessel from the right ventricle (*RV*). The gap (*short arrow*) between the left margin of the patch and the infundibular septum (*Inf S*) represents the residual ventricular septal defect.

The most common site for residual subpulmonary stenosis is the distal end of the patch (Fig. 38-6). The position of RV-PA conduits is variable enough that some improvisation may be necessary. However, the proximal (RV) end of the conduit can often be seen in a superiorly angulated subxiphoid long-axis view (L4 to L5) or a parasternal short-axis view. The distal end is usually best seen in a high parasternal short-axis view (Fig. 38-7). The midportion can usually be found by scanning up from the proximal end or down from the distal end.

Fig. 38-6. Parasternal short-axis view in a patient with repaired tetralogy of Fallot and residual pulmonary stenosis. The narrowest portion of the right ventricular outflow tract (*rvot*) is at the distal end of the rvot (*arrow*). Note the aneurysmal dilation of rvot. *ao* = aortic root; *mpa* = main pulmonary artery.

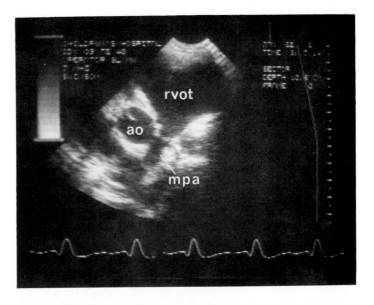

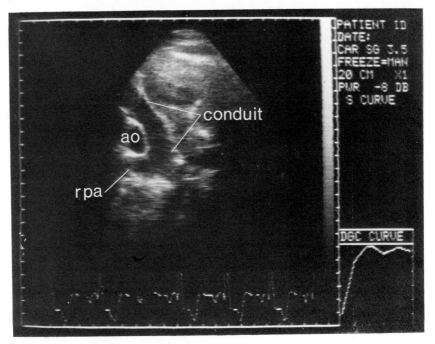

Fig. 38-7. High parasternal short-axis view of right ventricle to pulmonary artery conduit. *ao* = aortic root; *rpa* = right pulmonary artery.

CHAPTER 38. Evaluation of Postoperative Patients

TOTAL ANOMALOUS PULMONARY VENOUS CONNECTION
Anatomy

In supracardiac and infracardiac total anomalous pulmonary venous connection (TAPVC), the pulmonary venous (PV) confluence (horizontal and vertical channels, respectively) is anastomosed with the posterior LA wall and the connection with the systemic veins divided. The anastomosis is usually in the superior aspect of the posterior LA wall near the interatrial septum. TAPVC to the coronary sinus is usually repaired by unroofing the coronary sinus to create a connection with the LA and closing the usual orifice of coronary sinus in the right atrium (RA) with a patch. Total anomalous pulmonary venous connection to the RA (or proximal right superior vena cava) is usually repaired by baffling the PVs into the LA via an ASD (either naturally occurring or surgically created).

Examination Technique

The anastomosis between the PV confluence and the LA can be seen in subxiphoid long- and short-axis, apical 4-chamber, and parasternal long-axis views (Fig. 38-8A, B). The diameter of the anastomosis should be measured in at least two orthogonal planes and should approximate the diameter of the proximal PVs. If the diameter of the anastomosis is significantly smaller than that of the PV chamber in at least two views, then PV stenosis should be suspected. The sinus septal defect created between the coronary sinus and the LA can best be seen in subxiphoid short-axis views of the LA. The PV and LA often appear quite normal after repair of this lesion.

Fig. 38-8. (A) Subxiphoid 4-chamber (*left*) and short-axis (*right*) views in a patient with repaired total anomalous pulmonary venous connection. Note the large anastomosis between the pulmonary veins (*pv*) and the left atrium (*la*). (B) Subxiphoid 4-chamber (*left*) and short-axis (*right*) views in a patient with severe stenosis of the anastomosis between the pv and the la.

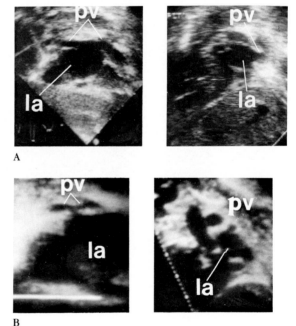

The baffle redirecting the PV blood to the LA in TAPVC to the RA is best observed in an apical 4-chamber view. The posterior aspect of the interatrial septum appears dense (patch material) and is directed more rightward than normal to incorporate the PVs. Disruption of the patch results in an ASD that can be seen from the apical or subxiphoid 4-chamber views.

Prosthetic Valves

Prosthetic valves can be examined with the same views used to examine the native valve in that position. Parasternal long- and short-axis views are particularly useful for examining aortic and mitral prostheses (Fig. 38-9). Prosthetic tricuspid valve can be examined by using apical 4-chamber views and by angling to the right from the parasternal long-axis views.

The information that can be derived depends on the type of prosthesis. In general, the following points should be addressed: (1) the motion of the occluder or leaflets, (2) the motion of the sewing ring with respect to surrounding cardiac tissue, and (3) valve-associated masses.

Fig. 38-9. Parasternal long-axis view shows a porcine bioprosthesis in the mitral position. The valve struts (*arrows*) project into the left ventricular cavity. *LA* = left atrium; *LV* = left ventricle; *RV* = right ventricle.

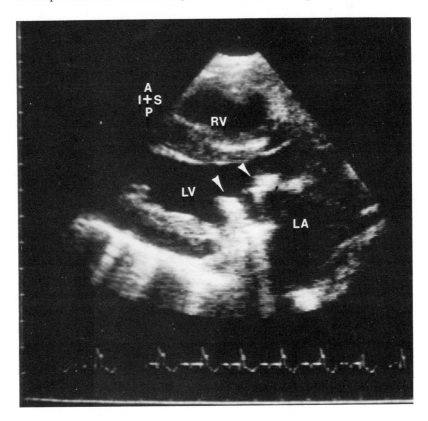

INTERATRIAL BAFFLES
Anatomy

Anatomic details of interatrial baffle repair of D-TGA and related lesions vary, depending on individual atrial characteristics as well as surgical technique. The systemic venous and PV pathways are difficult to represent in a flat, graphic approach because they have a complex, curved shape and do not lie in a single plane. In the Mustard repair, the superior and inferior venae cavae (SVC and IVC, respectively) pathways are directed leftward, toward the mitral valve. The two pathways lie superior and inferior to the PVs. The PV blood flow is directed anteriorly to the tricuspid orifice. In a sense, the systemic venous pathways form a partial doughnut, and the PV pathway forms a hole in the center of the atrial compartment. In the Senning repair, the SVC and IVC pathways are also directed leftward, but usually occupy a more central portion of the atrial compartment (i.e., the hole), while the PV pathway sweeps rightward, forming a partial doughnut as it proceeds from the more posterior PVs to the more anterior tricuspid valve. However, as seen in Figure 38-10A to D, there are more similarities than differences between these surgical procedures.

In the Mustard repair, the common sites of SVC and IVC obstruction are the entrance to the neo-RA and where the pathway sweeps around the PVs. Pulmonary venous obstruction occurs as a concentric narrowing in the middle of the atrium between the PVs posteriorly and the tricuspid valve anteriorly, due to encircling by the SVC and IVC pathways.

It is rare to encounter SVC or IVC obstruction in patients with the Senning repair. Pulmonary venous obstruction may occur at the midpoint of this pathway (the most rightward aspect) as it curves around the more centrally placed systemic venous pathway.

Diagnostic Echo Findings

In SVC obstruction, the combined findings of pathway narrowing or obliteration along its long axis and failure of contrast material to pass from the SVC to the RA on peripheral venous contrast injection are strong evidence for systemic venous obstruction. A dilated azygous vein is often visualized (subxiphoid S1), but is not specific for SVC obstruction. Dilation of the SVC may or may not be seen, depending on the adequacy of collaterals to the IVC.

Inferior vena caval obstruction is similar in appearance to SVC obstruction, although it is more awkward to obtain a contrast injection.

In the Mustard repair, PV obstruction occurs at the midatrium. From the subxiphoid S2 position, the PV pathway has an hour-glass configuration.

In the Senning repair, PV obstruction may occur as the pathway curves rightward, around the SVC pathway. The dimension of the pathway in this location should be measured in orthogonal planes (subxiphoid L2 and S2). The product of these dimensions is a sensitive indicator of obstruction. In both Mustard and Senning baffles, PV obstruction is accompanied by dilatation of the PVs and proximal PV changes.

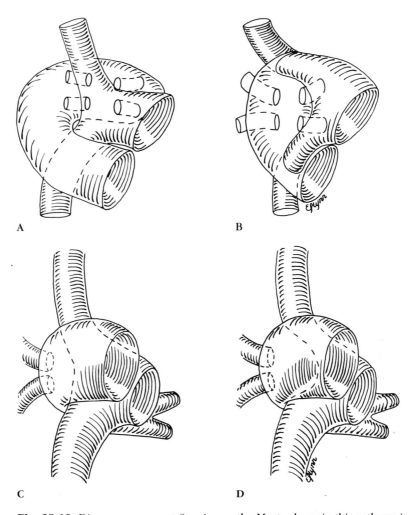

Fig. 38-10. Diagrams represent Senning repair (A) and Mustard repair (B) as seen from an anterior view. In the Senning repair, the systemic venous pathway is more centrally placed, while in the Mustard repair, this pathway is more leftward. Diagrams represent Senning repair (C) and Mustard repair (D) as viewed from a right lateral and slightly inferior position.

Examination Technique

In the Mustard and Senning baffles, the systemic venous pathways may be displayed in long axis by slight rotation (clockwise for SVC, counterclockwise for IVC) from the subxiphoid L2 position (Fig. 38-11A to C). This view also shows the far right portion of the PV pathway. In the Mustard repair, the same subxiphoid view displays the PV pathway in short axis as it occupies a central position within the atrial chamber.

In the Mustard repair, the length of the PV pathway usually runs anteroposterior (A-P) and therefore is seen in a straight transverse midatrial view (subxiphoid S2). In the Senning repair, the PV pathway is curved more rightward; its length is displayed from a subxiphoid long-axis (L2) or apical 4-chamber view (showing right-left coordinates), just inferior to the posi-

CHAPTER 38. Evaluation of Postoperative Patients

224

Fig. 38-11. (A) Subxiphoid long-axis view of atrium with clockwise rotation shows superior limb of systemic venous pathway in a patient with Senning repair. (B) Subxiphoid long-axis view of atrium with counterclockwise rotation shows inferior limb (*arrow*) of systemic venous pathway. The pulmonary venous atrium (*PVA*) is seen to either side of the systemic venous pathway. (C) Subxiphoid short-axis view through the systemic venous atrium at its connections with the superior vena cava (*svc*) and the inferior vena cava (*ivc*). *MV* = mitral valve; *pva* = pulmonary venous atrium; *RV* = right ventricle; *sva* = systemic venous atrium.

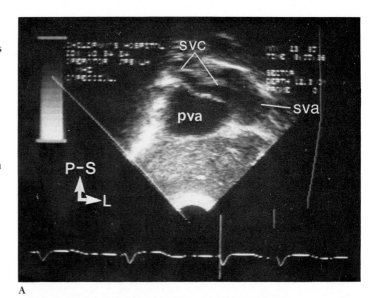

A

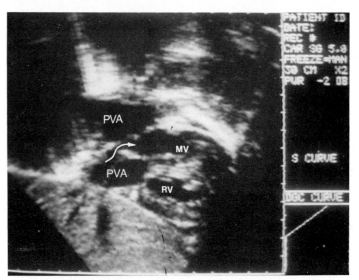

B

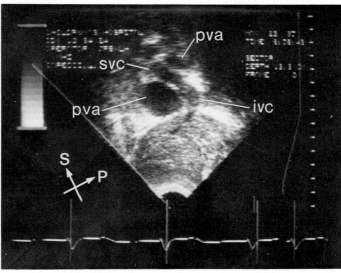

C

Fig. 38-12. (A) Subxiphoid 4-chamber view (L2) in a patient with Senning repair of D-transposition of the great arteries. The pulmonary venous atrium (*pva*) sweeps anteriorly around the right side of the centrally placed systemic venous atrium (*sva*). The narrowest portion of the pva is marked (*lines*). (B) Subxiphoid short-axis view of the extreme right extent of the pva. This view is orthogonal to that of Figure 38-12A. The usual site of pulmonary venous obstruction is denoted by the arrow. Subxiphoid long-axis (C) and short-axis (D) views of the pva in a patient with obstruction of the pulmonary venous pathway (*arrows*).

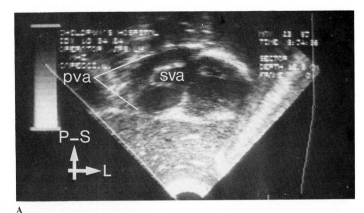

A

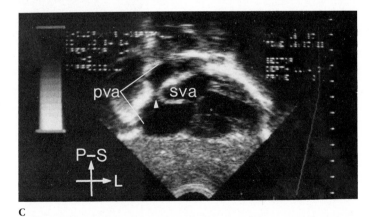

B

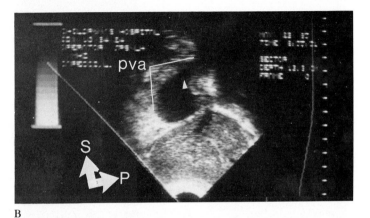

C

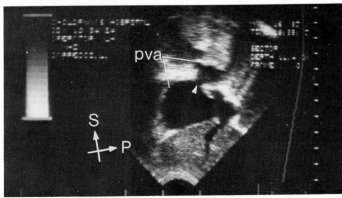

D

Fig. 38-13. Subxiphoid long-axis view shows residual defect (*arrow*) between the systemic venous atrium (*sva*) and pulmonary venous atrium (*pva*) following Senning operation.

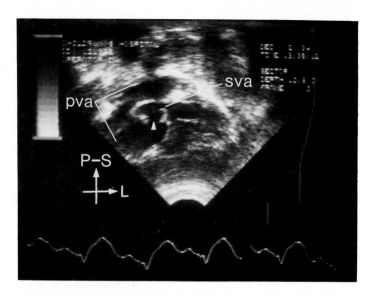

Fig. 38-14. Parasternal short-axis view of a patient with a pulmonary artery band. The bright echoes from the pulmonary artery band are seen as it constricts the proximal main pulmonary artery. The diameter of the constricted area can be compared with the pulmonary or aortic annulus diameter. *pa* = pulmonary artery.

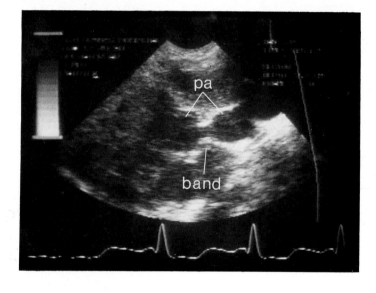

tion from which the SVC pathway is displayed (Fig. 38-12A). Viewing the PV pathway in the orthogonal transverse plane (approximately subxiphoid S2) allows measurement of the PV chamber as it passes behind the SVC pathway (Fig. 38-12B). Both views must be visualized in evaluating the patient with pulmonary venous obstruction (Fig. 38-12C, D).

Residual interatrial septal defects following the Senning repair can often be seen using subxiphoid (Fig. 38-13) or apical views. Since the direction of flow is almost invariably from the systemic venous to the PV atrium, a peripheral vein contrast injection is extremely useful for documenting residual interatrial communications.

Pitfalls

The systemic venous pathways usually narrow relative to the PV pathway and may curve out of the sector plane, giving a false impression of complete pathway obstruction. In addition, there are no absolute criteria for the degree of narrowing consistent with hemodynamically significant obstruction.

The Mustard repair, the area of PV obstruction, is a concentric constriction. In the Senning repair, the narrowest point of the PV pathway may be elliptic and therefore must be evaluated in orthogonal planes.

PULMONARY ARTERY BAND

The PA band is seen as a constriction of the lumen of the PA. The area is encircled by brightly reflective echoes. The band is best seen in high parasternal or subxiphoid (S4) views that provide a longitudinal view of the main pulmonary artery (MPA) if it is positioned anteriorly (Fig. 38-14). If the PA is posterior to the aorta, a subxiphoid long-axis view with superior angulation from the 4-chamber position will often best display the MPA segment.

The efficacy of a PA band has been related to the diameter of the constriction as an absolute number or in comparison to the pulmonary or aortic annulus. Although this measurement is helpful, variables such as echo beam with angle of interrogation and artifacts related to intense reflections of the band material are problems. Moreover, associated problems such as aortic outflow obstruction and A-V valve regurgitation may affect pulmonary band effectiveness, regardless of the degree of obstruction. At the present time, Doppler estimation of band gradient, utilizing the Bernoulli equation, is a more effective method for assessing band adequacy, while visualization of the band area offers supportive evidence of the degree of constriction and direct data concerning the position of the band.

BIBLIOGRAPHY

Andrade, J. L., Serino, W., De Leval, M., et al. Two-dimensional echocardiographic assessment of surgically closed ventricular septal defect. *Am. J. Cardiol.* 52:325, 1983.

Aziz, K. U., Paul, M. H., and Bharati, S. Two dimensional echocardiographic evaluation of Mustard operation for D-transposition of the great arteries. *Am. J. Cardiol.* 47:654, 1981.

Canale, J. M., Sahn, D. J., Copeland, J. G., et al. Two-dimensional Doppler echocardiographic/M-mode echocardiographic and phonocardiographic method for study of extracardiac heterograft valved conduits in the right ventricular outflow tract position. *Am. J. Cardiol.* 49:93, 1982.

Chin, A. J., Sanders, S. P., Williams, R. G., et al. Two-dimensional echocardiographic assessment of caval and pulmonary venous pathways after the Senning operation. *Am. J. Cardiol.* 52:118, 1983.

Foale, R. A., King, M. E., Gordon, D., et al. Pseudoaneurysm of the pulmonary artery after the banding procedure: Two-dimensional echocardiographic description. *J. Am. Coll. Cardiol.* 3:371, 1984.

Index

Index

Absent pulmonary valve syndrome, with
    tetralogy of Fallot, 163–164
Anomalous pulmonary venous
    connection
  partial, 84–85
  total, 74–82
    anatomy of, 74
    diagnostic echo findings in, 74
      indirect, 74
    diagnostic problems, 82
    examination technique, 77–81
    postoperative evaluation of,
      220–221
    superior vena cava and, 75
    suprasternal notch view of, 77
Aorta
  ascending
    in great artery D-transposition, 166,
      167
    right parasternal view of, 8
  atresia
    in hypoplastic left heart syndrome,
      121–126
  coarctation of. See Coarctation of the
    aorta
  descending, 197
  echo displays of, 8
  left, 8
  right, 8
  in tetralogy of Fallot, 159
Aortic arch
  atresia of, 149
  high right parasternal view of, 9
  in hypoplastic left heart syndrome,
    122
  interrupted, 146–149
    anatomy of, 146
    diagnostic echo findings in,
      146–148
    diagnostic problems in, 148–149
    examination technique in, 148
    in truncus arteriosus, 186
  right
    parasternal view of, 9
    subxiphoid long-axis view of,
      160
  suprasternal notch view of, 27–28,
    145
  transducer position for, 27
  tubular hypoplasia of, 144
Aortic valve
  bicuspid vs. tricuspid, 139, 141
  examination technique in, 4, 6,
    141
  fluttering of, 130
  herniation of, 62

Aortic valve—*Continued*
  in left ventricular outflow obstruc-
    tion, 127
  prosthetic, 221
  stenosis of, 137–141
    2-D examination of, 141
    anatomy of, 137
    diagnostic echo findings in,
      137–139
      indirect, 140
    diagnostic problems in, 141
    examination technique in, 141
    M-mode examination of, 141
Aorticopulmonary window, 86–87
Atresia
  aorta. *See* Aortic arch, atresia of
  pulmonary. *See* Pulmonary atresia
  tricuspid. *See* Tricuspid atresia
Atrial appendages
  high transverse parasternal view of,
    209
  juxtaposition of, 208–210
  normal anatomy of, 208
Atrial septal defect, 36–50
  anatomy of, 36–37
  coronary sinus, 37
  diagnostic echo findings in, 37
    indirect, 37
  examination technique in, 37–48
    pitfalls, 49–50
  false-positive diagnosis of, 49
  positions of, 36
  postoperative evaluation of, 214–216
  primum-type, 36
    subxiphoid 4-chamber view of, 43
    viewing positions, 42
  repair of
    anatomy of, 214
    examination technique, 214–216
    postoperative evaluation of,
      214–216
  secundum-type, 36, 40, 41
    false-positive diagnosis of, 49
  septum primum in, 37, 39
  sinus venosus-type, 36
    inferior, 47
    superior, 46
Atrioventricular canal defect
  complete, 63–70
    anatomy of, 63–64
    diagnostic echo findings in, 64–68
    diagnostic problems in, 70
    lesions associated with, 64, 195
    Rastelli type C, 65, 67
    surgical repair of, 63–64, 214, 215
    truncus arteriosus and, 186

Atrioventricular septal defect. *See* Atrioventricular canal defect
Atrioventricular valves
  apical 4-chamber view of, 11
  in double inlet single ventricle, 201
  double outlet right ventricle and, 180
  leaflets, 45
  long-axis views of, 31
  number of, 195
  in single ventricle, 202
  straddling, 204–207
Atrium
  appendages. *See* Atrial appendages
  left. *See* Left atrium
  right. *See* Right atrium
  right-to-left shunting, in tricuspid atresia, 101
Azygous vein
  parasternal parasagittal view of, 195
  subxiphoid parasagittal view of, 191

Brachiocephalic vessels, right parasternal view of, 9
Bulboventricular foramen, 199, 200

Cardiomyopathy, hypertrophic. *See* Hypertrophic cardiomyopathy
Cardiovascular disease, complex, 187–212
Carotid arteries, aortic arch interruption between, 146, 147
Carotid pulse recordings, in hypertrophic cardiomyopathy, 135
Coarctation of the aorta, 142–145
  anatomy of, 142
  congenital mitral obstruction and, 113
  diagnostic echo findings in, 142
  diagnostic problems in, 144
  double outlet right ventricle and, 180
  examination technique in, 142
  in hypoplastic left heart syndrome, 121
  vs. interrupted aortic arch, 149
  patent ductus arteriosus in, 145
  suprasternal notch view of, 143, 144
Congenital heart defects, segmental diagnostic approach to, 188–197
Congenital mitral obstruction. *See* Mitral valve, congenital obstruction of
Conotruncal abnormalities, 151–186
  anatomy of, 152–154
  congenital mitral obstruction and, 113

Conotruncal abnormalities—*Continued*
  general features of, 152–154
  interrupted aortic arch and, 146
  mitral valve straddling and, 207
  ventricular septal defects in, 51
Conotruncus, examination of, 197
Conus, abnormal development of, 152
Cor triatriatum, 118–119
  anatomy of, 118
  vs. congenital mitral obstruction, 113
  diagnostic echo findings in, 118
  diagnostic problems in, 119
  examination technique in, 119
Coronary artery
  left, anomalous, 89–91
Coronary sinus
  apical 4-chamber view of, 12
  atrial septal defect and, 37, 48
  dilated, vs. juxtapositioned right atrial appendage, 210
  low subxiphoid 4-chamber view of, 49

Dextrocardia, 211–212
Double outlet right ventricle. *See* Right ventricle, double outlet

Ebstein's anomaly, of tricuspid valve, 94–98
  anatomy of, 94
  diagnostic echo findings in, 95–98
  diagnostic problems in, 98
  examination technique in, 98
Eustachian valve, vs. interatrial septum, 190

Foramen ovale
  multiple perforations of, 50

Great arteries
  anteroposterior position of, 165
  aorticopulmonary window and, 87
  corrected transposition of, 170–176
    anatomy of, 170
    diagnostic echo findings in, 170–176
    diagnostic problems in, 176
    examination technique in, 176
    great artery position in, 175
    hand rule in, 175, 176
    lesions associated with, 170
    papillary muscle pattern in, 174
    trabecular muscle pattern in, 174
    ventricular identity in, 172
    ventricular shape in, 174

Index

Great arteries—*Continued*
  in double outlet right ventricle, 178
  D-transposition of, 165–169
    anatomy of, 165–166, 222
    atrioventricular straddling and, 207
    diagnostic echo findings in, 166,
      167, 222
    diagnostic problems in, 169
    examination technique in,
      166–169
    left juxtaposition of atrial append-
      ages in, 209
    left ventricle outflow obstruction
      in, 127, 131
    patent ductus arteriosus and, 71
    postoperative evaluation of,
      222–227
    Senning repair of, 225
    tricuspid atresia and, 99
    ventriculoarterial alignment in,
      165
  examination of, 197
  L-transposition of. *See* Great arteries,
    corrected transposition of
  simple transposition of. *See* D-trans-
    position of
  ventricular origin of, 153

Hand rule, of great artery transposition,
    175–176
Heart
  apical approach, 11–13
  interrelationships of different views,
    29–33
  malpositions of, 211–212
  parasternal approach, 4–13
  precordial imaging of, 4–13
    long-axis view, 4, 5
    right, 8–10
    short-axis view, 4, 6, 7
  subxiphoid approach, 14–26
    long-axis planes, 16, 17, 20, 21, 25
    orthogonal plane, 24
    short-axis views, 22
    transducer positions for, 14–15
  suprasternal approach, 27–28
Heterotaxy syndrome, 188–197
  atrioventricular canal in, 195
  conotruncus in, 197
  great arteries in, 197
  venoatrial segment, 188–193
  ventricles in, 196
Hypertension, pulmonary. *See* Pulmo-
    nary hypertension
Hypertrophic cardiomyopathy,
    132–135

Hypertrophic cardiomyopathy—*Cont.*
  anatomy of, 132
  carotid-pulse recordings in, 135
  diagnostic echo findings in, 132–134
    indirect, 135
  diagnostic problems in, 135
  examination technique in, 135
  M-mode recordings in, 135
  short-segment obstruction in, 130
Hypoplastic left heart syndrome,
    121–126
  anatomy of, 121
  aortic atresia in, 121–126
  diagnostic echo findings in, 123–126
  diagnostic problems in, 126
  examination technique in, 126
  mitral atresia in, 121–126
  variations in, 126
Hypoplastic right heart syndrome,
    103–107
  anatomy of, 103
  diagnostic echo findings in, 103–107
  diagnostic problems in, 107
  examination technique in, 107

Infundibular septum
  in double outlet right ventricle, 178
  in double-chambered right ventricle,
    108
  posterior malalignment of, 129
  in tetralogy of Fallot, 152, 155, 157
Infundibulum, abnormal development
    of, 152
Interatrial baffles
  anatomy of, 222
  diagnostic echo findings in, 222
  examination technique, 223–227
  Mustard repair of transposition, 223
  postoperative evaluation of, 222–227
  Senning repair of transposition, 223
Interatrial septum
  vs. eustachian valve, 190
  right parasternal view of, 8
  subxiphoid 4-chamber view of, 24
  subxiphoid approach to, 18, 38
  in tricuspid atresia, 102
Interventricular septum
  apical 4-chamber view of, 11
  atrioventricular valve straddling of,
    204–207
  in great artery D-transposition, 166
  in hypertrophic cardiomyopathy, 132
  in hypoplastic right heart syndrome,
    103–107
  malalignment-type defect of, 127
  parasternal long-axis view of, 4, 5

Index

Interventricular septum—*Continued*
  parasternal short-axis view of, 4, 7
  transverse parasternal view of, 7

Left atrium
  apical 4-chamber view of, 11
  in congenital mitral obstruction, 113
  cor triatriatum and, 118
  parasternal short-axis view of, 4, 6
  subxiphoid long-axis view of, 16, 18
Left ventricle
  apical 2-chamber view of, 30
  apical 4-chamber view of, 11
  in congenital mitral obstruction, 113
  double outlet, vs. tetralogy of Fallot,
    156, 161
  in great artery L-transposition, 171
  in hypertrophic obstructive car-
    diomyopathy, 133
  hypoplastic, 121–126
    apical 4-chamber view of, 196
  inflow
    subxiphoid long-axis view, 16
    viewing interrelationships, 31
  long-axis view of, 29–30
  outflow tract
    anteroposterior coordinates of,
      130
    apical 2-chamber view of, 12
    fixed obstruction of, 127–131
      anatomy of, 127
      diagnostic echo findings in,
        128–129
        indirect, 130
      diagnostic problems in, 130–131
      examination technique in, 130
    in great artery D-transposition, 166
    in great artery L-transposition, 172,
      173
    in hypertrophic cardiomyopathy,
      134
    obstruction of
      congenital mitral stenosis and,
        117
    parasternal short-axis view of, 4
    short-axis views of, 33
    subxiphoid long-axis view of, 44,
      123
    subxiphoid short-axis view of, 156
    in tetralogy of Fallot, 59
  papillary muscles of, 174
  parasternal views of, 7, 30, 32–33
    right, 8–10
  single, 199
    with l-ventricular loop, 200, 201

Left ventricle—*Continued*
  subxiphoid long-axis view of, 20
    in congenital mitral obstruction,
      116
  subxiphoid short-axis view of, 25, 44
    in great artery transposition, 168
  subxiphoid view of, 126
  tricuspid valve straddling and, 204,
    206
  viewing interrelationships, 29–30
    long axis, 29–30
    short axis, 32–33

Mesocardia, 212
Mitral valve
  apical 4-chamber view of, 196
  atresia, 121–126
  congenital obstruction of, 113–117
    anatomy of, 113
    classic parachute, 113
      in great artery transposition, 174
    diagnostic echo findings in,
      114–117
    supportive findings in, 117
  in cor triatriatum, 119
  doming of, 114
  hypoplasia, 196
  in hypoplastic left heart syndrome,
    121–126
  M-mode echo findings, 114
  parasternal short-axis view of, 4, 6, 7
  prosthetic, 221
  straddling, 204–207
Mustard operation
  in interatrial baffles, 223, 225
  pitfalls, 227

Patent ductus arteriosus, 71–73
  anatomy of, 71
  diagnostic echo findings in, 71
  diagnostic problems in, 72
  examination technique, 72
  high parasagittal parasternal view of,
    72
  in hypoplastic left heart syndrome,
    121
  in hypoplastic right heart syndrome,
    103
  subxiphoid short-axis view of, 73
  suprasternal notch view of, 71
Postoperative patients, evaluation of,
  214–227
Prosthetic valves, 221
Pulmonary artery
  bifurcation of, 167

Index

Pulmonary artery—*Continued*
Doppler examination of, 103
in great artery transposition, 167
in hypoplastic right heart syndrome,
103–107
main
in absent pulmonary valve syndrome, 163
in interrupted aortic arch, 148
suprasternal notch view of, 148
in truncus arteriosus, 185
parasternal short-axis view of, 4, 6
right
parasternal view of, 8, 9
subxiphoid long-axis view of, 23
suprasternal notch view of, 28
stenosis of, 103–107
in tetralogy of Fallot, 158
Pulmonary artery band, postoperative
evaluation of, 227
Pulmonary artery pressure, in great artery transposition, 168
Pulmonary atresia
diagnostic problems in, 107
in hypoplastic right heart syndrome,
103–107
vs. tricuspid stenosis, 107
Pulmonary valve
absent, 163–164
in double-chambered right ventricle,
110
in hypoplastic right heart syndrome,
103
M-mode echo findings, 110
patent vs. atretic, 107
root, size of, 110
stenosis of, 111–112
anatomy of, 111
diagnostic echo findings in, 111
diagnostic problems in, 112
double-chambered right ventricle
and, 108
examination technique in, 111
high transverse parasternal view of,
112
subxiphoid short-axis view of,
112
Pulmonary veins
anomalous connection. *See* Anomalous pulmonary venous
connection
cor triatriatum and, 118
juxtaposition of atrial appendages
and, 208

Rhabdomyoma, vs. hypertrophic cardiomyopathy, 135
Right atrium
apical 4-chamber view of, 11
subxiphoid long-axis view of, 16
Right ventricle
apical 4-chamber view of, 11
chirality of, 175
dilation, pulmonary regurgitation
and, 163
double chambered, 108–110
anatomy of, 108
diagnostic echo findings in, 108
indirect, 110
diagnostic problems in, 110
Doppler examination of, 110
examination technique in, 110
lesions associated with, 110
double outlet, 178–183
anatomy of, 178–180
anomalies associated with, 180
complete atrioventricular defect
and, 64
diagnostic echo findings in,
180–182
diagnostic problems, 183
examination technique in, 182
mitral valve straddling in, 207
vs. tetralogy of Fallot, 155
ventricular septal defect in, 51
hypoplasia of, 103–107
inflow
subxiphoid long-axis view of, 20
tricuspid valve straddling and, 204
outflow tract
in great artery L-transposition, 172,
173
in hypoplastic right heart syndrome, 103
obstruction, vs. double-chambered
right ventricle, 110
parasternal short-axis view of, 4, 6,
101
patency of, 161
subxiphoid view of, 25, 101
in tetralogy of Fallot, 156, 157
in tricuspid atresia, 99
in truncus arteriosus, 186
parasternal short-axis view of
in hypoplastic right heart syndrome, 107
in pulmonary valve deformity, 107
pulmonary atresia and, 103
pulmonary stenosis and, 103

Index

Right ventricle—*Continued*
  single, 199
  subxiphoid long-axis view of, 125

Senning operation, 223, 225–227
Septum. *See specific location*
Shunt lesions, 35–91
Situs inversus, subxiphoid view of, 189
Situs solitus, subxiphoid view of, 189
Splenic dysgenesis syndrome, double
    outlet right ventricle and, 180
Stenosis. *See specific location*
Subaortic stenosis
  anatomy of, 127
  apical 2-chamber view of, 129
  congenital mitral obstruction and,
    113
  diagnostic difficulties, 130
  fibromuscular, 130
  parasternal long-axis view of, 128
  subxiphoid long-axis view of, 128
Subpulmonary stenosis
  in great artery transposition, 169
  tetralogy of Fallot and, 218
Supravalvar aortic stenosis, parasternal
    view of, 8
Supravalvar mitral ring
  vs. cor triatriatum, 119
  subxiphoid 4-chamber view of, 115
  subxiphoid long-axis view of, 114

Tetralogy of Fallot, 155–161
  absent pulmonary valve syndrome
    and, 163–164
  anatomy of, 155–156, 216
  complete atrioventricular defect and,
    64
  diagnostic echo findings in, 156–160
  diagnostic problems in, 161
  vs. double-chambered right ventricle,
    110
  double-chambered right ventricle
    and, 108
  examination techniques in, 161, 217
  infundibular septal shift in, 152
  left ventricle outflow tract in, 59
  mild, 157
  postoperative evaluation of, 216–219
  right ventricle outflow tract in, 156,
    157, 161
  severe, 157
  vs. truncus arteriosus, 186
  variations of, 160
  ventricular septal defect in, 51

Total anomalous pulmonary venous
    connection
  anatomy of, 74
  diagnostic echo findings in, 74
    indirect, 74
  diagnostic problems, 82
  examination technique, 77–81
  postoperative evaluation of, 220–221
  superior vena cava and, 75
Tricuspid atresia, 99–102
  anatomy of, 99
  apical 4-chamber view of, 100, 101
  atrial appendages juxtaposition in,
    209
  diagnostic echo findings in, 100–101
  diagnostic problems in, 102
  examination technique in, 101
Tricuspid valve
  Ebstein's anomaly of, 94–98
    anatomy of, 94
    apical 4-chamber view of, 95
    diagnostic echo findings in, 95–98
    diagnostic problems in, 98
    examination technique in, 98
    severe form of, 97
    in great artery L-transposition, 171
  hypoplastic annulus, 102
  in hypoplastic right heart syndrome,
    103
  stenosis of, in pulmonary atresia, 107
  straddling, 204–207
    in ventricular septal defect, 62
  subxiphoid long-axis view of, 20
  systolic fluttering of, 53
Truncus arteriosus, 184–186
  anatomy of, 184
  diagnostic echo findings in, 184
  diagnostic problems in, 186
  examination technique in, 184
  lesions associated with, 186

Valsalva maneuver, in hypertrophic car-
    diomyopathy, 135
Valvar aortic stenosis. *See* Aortic valve,
    stenosis of
Vena cava
  inferior, subxiphoid views of, 17, 208
  superior
    atrial septal defect and, 48
    azygous vein connection to, 195
    bilateral, 194
    connections, 192
    left suprasternal notch short-axis
      view of, 194
    right parasternal view of, 8

Index

Ventricle(s)
  identification of, in great artery trans-
      position, 172
  left. *See* Left ventricle
  morphology of, 196
  number of, 196
  right. *See* Right ventricle
  single, 199–202
      anatomy of, 199
      diagnostic echo findings in, 199
      double-inlet, 200, 201
      examination techniques in,
          200–202
      interrupted aortic arch and, 146
      left, 199
      right, 199
      subxiphoid short-axis view of, 202
Ventricular septal defect, 51–62, 199
  anatomy of, 51–52, 216
  anterior malalignment type, 51
      diagnostic echo findings in, 53
  vs. aorticopulmonary window, 86
  atrioventricular saddling and, 204,
      205
  A-V canal type, 51
      diagnostic echo findings in, 53
  congenital mitral obstruction and,
      113
  conoventricular, 51
  diagnostic echo findings in, 52–53
      indirect, 53–54

Ventricular septal defect—*Continued*
  diagnostic problems in, 61
  examination techniques in, 54–61,
      217
  inlet, 51
  interrupted aortic arch and, 146
  intracristal, 51
  left-to-right shunting in, 53
  malalignment type, 59
  multiple small, 53
  muscular, 52
      diagnostic echo findings in, 53
      parasternal long-axis view of, 61
  parasternal long-axis view of, 54
  patching of, 214
      subxiphoid 4-chamber view of,
          215
  perimembranous, 51
      diagnostic echo findings in, 52–53
      subxiphoid long-axis view of, 56
      subxiphoid short-axis view of, 57
  posterior malalignment type, 51
      diagnostic echo findings in, 53
  postoperative evaluation of, 216–219
  subaortic, 51
  subaortic outflow, 51
  subpulmonary, 51
      subxiphoid short-axis view of, 60
  "Swiss-cheese," 53
  in tetralogy of Fallot, 159
  trabecular, 53

Index